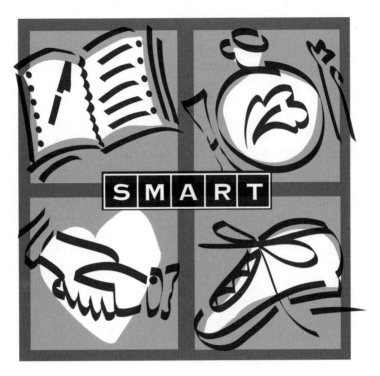

CHOICES for Health ™

Written by:

Sandy Seiler Miller, MS, RD, LD

Edited by:

Suzanne Girard Eberle, MS, RD

Special Contributions from:

Nancy Becker, MS, RD, LD; Bonnie Bissell, MA, LPC; Nessa Elila, MA, LPC;
Nancie Fisher, RD; Susan Landgren, MS, RD, LD; Cathy Seeber, RD, LD

Workbook Reviewers:

Marilyn Frankel, MA; Michael Girard; Katherine Keniston; Kennan Kuffel;
Shannon Stember, RD, LD; Julia Surtshin, MS Ed; Birgitta von Schlumperger, PhD

A Bit of History

Encouraging people to make personal choices for a healthier lifestyle has been the cornerstone of Providence Health System's weight management program since its inception in 1982. The original program, titled *Weighing the CHOICES*, received an Outstanding Community Health Promotion Program Award from the U.S. Department of Health and Human Services in 1986. After numerous updates, the program evolved into the *CHOICES* program in 1994. With new information and the shared experiences of thousands of participants, revisions were undertaken again in 1999 and *Smart CHOICES for Health*™ emerged from the *CHOICES* program. This workbook is the product of this evolution.

This book is dedicated to the thousands of Oregonians who have participated in this program. Many thanks for their wisdom and experience. It is also dedicated to the Providence Health System instructors (dietitians, mental health professionals and fitness specialists) who have enriched the program with their expertise and their caring commitment to the health and wellness of others.

Smart CHOICES for Health™

Cover Design: Marcia Barrentine

Interior Design & Production: Heidi Bay

ISBN 0-9672735-3-6

For information, write:
Attn: *Smart CHOICES* Program
Providence Resource Line
Tigard Business Center
11308 SW 68th Parkway, Suite 125
Tigard, OR 97223

For ordering information, see the order form located on the back page of this workbook.

Disclaimer: Consult your physician or primary health care provider before undertaking the changes in diet, exercise or other health behaviors suggested in *Smart CHOICES*. This is especially important if you have a medical problem such as diabetes, high blood pressure or heart disease. If you are experiencing psychological distress or have a history of psychological difficulties, you should consult with a licensed mental health professional before embarking in this program. For additional guidance and support, a registered dietitian's counsel is recommended.

Providence Health System and the program's developer, Sandy Miller, assume no responsibility or liability for personal or other injury, loss, or damage that may result from the suggestions or information in this publication.

Table of Contents

Welcome to
Smart CHOICES for Health™

Congratulations! Just opening this book shows you care about your health or at least are curious about learning more about your health. The road to a healthier lifestyle can be full of potholes and detours. It's easy to get sidetracked. The *Smart CHOICES for Health*™ program helps you navigate obstacles and gain the necessary skills to keep you headed in the right direction. It's a personal road map, allowing you to travel at your own pace and in a way that suits your needs.

A healthy lifestyle doesn't happen by accident. It's all about making smart choices. These choices don't have to be giant steps like becoming a vegetarian or training for a marathon. In fact, making too many changes all at once often leads to giving up. The power of *Smart CHOICES* lies in making *smaller* changes *over time*. Like turning the TV off and going for a walk. Deciding on a bean burrito instead of a double cheeseburger for lunch. Or satisfying a craving for chocolate with a small piece instead of depriving yourself.

Small changes, the ones you make day to day, add up in the long run. You may not completely change a lifetime of habits and patterns your first time through the *Smart CHOICES* program. You will, however, have an opportunity to try out many powerful tools and skills. Try them on for size. See what fits and decide which ones work for you. Everyone's path to a healthier weight is unique. Finding the right approach is often a matter of trial and error. Ultimately, you'll gain a repertoire of powerful skills that will guide you for a lifetime.

The Difference between *Smart CHOICES* and Other Diet Methods

When it comes to losing weight, many people try one diet after another. The problem with diets is that they don't work. If you go *on* a diet, eventually at some point you go *off* the diet. Since diets don't encourage you to make permanent changes, you return to your old habits and your old weight. The *Smart CHOICES* program encourages lifestyle changes (not diets) that you can stick with, not for a day, or a week, but for a lifetime. That's what it takes to lose weight and keep it off permanently.

Smart CHOICES is based on self-awareness activities and personalized weekly plans which you design for yourself. Over the next ten weeks, you'll discover what works best for YOU to reach and maintain a healthy weight. The chart on the following page depicts the major differences between *Smart CHOICES* and other weight loss methods.

Smart CHOICES	OTHER DIET METHODS
A Non-dieting approach: • Encourages you to eat by listening to internal cues of hunger and satiety, not external food plans or diets. • No lists of "good" foods and "bad" foods. All food is acceptable.	**Diet approach:** • Prepackaged foods or supplements. • Rigid food plan based on a set number of calories or grams of fat.
Encourages an active lifestyle: • No specified exercise or activities; recognizes all forms of movement. • Self-paced. • Encourages you to listen to your body.	**Rigid exercise plan:** • Not flexible; doesn't meet individual needs. • Promotes a "no pain, no gain" philosophy.
Personalized plan for change: • Personalized weekly plans direct your journey towards a healthier weight.	**Inflexible plan:** • "One size fits all" mandates.
Emphasizes self-empowerment and self-responsibility: • Promotes personal choices and options. • Focuses on "skill power" vs. willpower. • Encourages problem-solving and developing solutions that are right for you. • Encourages a "take charge" attitude.	**Promotes dependency:** • Dictates what to do and how to do it. • Encourages a dependent relationship with the program for continued success.
Acknowledges that healthy bodies come in a range of weights, shapes and sizes: • Recognizes that people of all sizes and shapes can improve their health and energy level through a healthier lifestyle.	**Set standards for weight and size:** • Promotes an "ideal" body size, shape or weight. • Doesn't account for personal differences.
Encourages long-term lifestyle changes: • Recommends slow, gradual weight loss — weight that stays off!	**Promises a quick-fix:** • Short term, prescribed diet promoting a quick weight loss.

Getting Started

Change is a process, not an event. *Smart CHOICES* helps you make changes gradually according to your tastes, needs and current lifestyle. This workbook will guide you from week to week. You'll experiment with new tools and techniques designed to help you improve your health and lose weight permanently. Try them on for size. See how they feel. Explore your options. Keep what works for you and discard the rest.

This Week You Will Learn:

- The nuts and bolts of the *Smart CHOICES* program.
- How to use this workbook.
- How to assess your readiness for change.
- Ways to measure your progress.
- How to plan for fitness.
- The value of record keeping.

Program Content

Smart CHOICES is a ten-week program designed to help you develop skills in four key areas: Food/nutrition, Fitness, Emotional support, S.M.A.R.T. planning.

Learn how to make healthier food choices, design and stick with an exercise program, and talk yourself through the rough times. Once and for all, you'll have the knowledge and the tools you need to make permanent lifestyle changes.

Food/Nutrition

Smart CHOICES will help you manage your weight without diets, pills, formulas or special food combinations. You won't find any lists of "good" foods or "bad" foods. Instead, you'll discover how to eat based on your body's internal feelings of hunger. You won't need external food plans or diets. You'll enjoy the foods you love without feeling deprived. At the same time, you'll learn to honor your body's hunger/fullness signals and nutritional needs.

Fitness

No early-morning calisthenics or expensive gym memberships; *Smart CHOICES* simply encourages you to move more. You decide how to accomplish this goal. *Smart CHOICES* coaches you every step of the way. You'll get in shape to do the things you want to do — keep up with your grandchildren or complete a day-long hike.

Emotional Support

To build a new lifestyle, you need a strong support system. *Smart CHOICES* helps you identify areas where you may need support and teaches you how to effectively ask others for help. You'll also tune in to the connection between food and feelings, learn to be positive when you talk to yourself, and become more accepting of your body.

S.M.A.R.T. Planning

You can't make important lifestyle changes — eating healthier, being more physically active and garnering emotional support — without planning. Planning is the foundation of the *Smart CHOICES* program. Establishing a plan gives you motivation and direction. Each week you'll make a S.M.A.R.T. (Specific, Measurable, Achievable, Relevant, Trackable) plan to help direct your actions and to serve as your personal road map to success.

Note: The *Smart CHOICES* program is designed to be repeated until you master the skills that you need.

Guidelines for Using this Workbook

1. What to expect.

Each week you will find the following sections in your workbook:

- **Introduction** — Alerts you to the topics covered each week.

- **Reflections** — Gives you an opportunity at the beginning of each week to take a few minutes to reflect over the previous week. You can hone in on any helpful insights that you uncovered, such as personal successes and challenges.

- **Facts of Life** — Provides a chance to pause and rethink some old stumbling blocks in a new and enlightening way.

- **Skill Practice** — At the end of each chapter you will find several suggested activities to try in the upcoming week. The purpose of this weekly homework is to give you the opportunity to practice new skills and develop new habits that will help you lose weight and keep it off permanently.

2. Complete one chapter each week.

Your *Smart CHOICES* workbook contains ten chapters to be completed in ten weeks. You may choose to take longer than ten weeks; you set the pace. You'll benefit the most, however, by setting aside some time EACH week, just as if you were attending a class. Expect to spend approximately one hour on each week's lesson. Be certain to work through the chapters (weeks) in the order they appear. For example, week one contains chapter one.

Each week you'll find all four core components (food, fitness, emotional support and planning) represented to varying degrees. To get you started, the early weeks provide a great deal of information on nutrition and exercise. The remaining weeks supply a mixture of information and activities dealing with food, fitness and emotional support. Planning or record-keeping opportunities appear every week.

3. Be an active participant.

To benefit fully from the *Smart CHOICES* program, don't just read through your workbook. Grab a pencil and complete the activities. There are several sections in this workbook in which you participate:

- **Hands-on Activities** — Hands-on activities give you a chance to practice and apply the information presented each week. Passing over these activities in order to keep reading defeats the purpose of this workbook. Neglecting to complete the activities robs you of valuable opportunities to learn and improve on vital new skills.

- **FOOD & ACTIVITY JOURNAL** — Record in this journal on a regular basis, each week tracking exercise and a different aspect of your eating routine. Keeping this journal helps you become more aware of your personal habits. It also provides a means of monitoring your progress so you can recognize and acknowledge your successes.

- **S.M.A.R.T. Plans** — Design and complete weekly S.M.A.R.T. plans based on goals that are Specific, Measurable, Achievable, Relevant and Trackable. You will have specific directions or instructions at your fingertips to help you stay on track.

4. Honor your commitment.

No one expects you to be perfect. Honor your commitment to make lifelong changes by doing the best you can. Of course, you may choose not to do every activity or assignment. It's up to you. As with many things in life, you gain the most when you invest the most. Make the effort with *Smart CHOICES*. Achieving a healthy weight and feeling your best — what could be more important than that?

5. Refer to the Appendix for extra resources.

There are many helpful tools in this section:

- CALORIE & FAT COUNTER

- Meal and snack ideas (including quick-fix dinner recipes)

- Resources (books, videos, websites)

- Blank forms (FOOD & ACTIVITY JOURNAL, Food Guide Pyramid, worksheets)

Are You Ready for Change?

With behavior change, there is no such thing as failure. Change occurs on a continuum; sometimes we leap, sometimes we crawl and sometimes we slip back...

—*Michael Samuelson*

Change Happens in Stages

It's unrealistic to expect that habits, ingrained over the years, will be shed overnight. Changing a behavior is a process, not a decision. It takes time and happens in stages. Researchers have found that successful self-changers unconsciously follow a sequence of activities and attitudes when they make behavior changes. As you read through the stages of change outlined below, think about a habit that you are interested in changing.

Stages of Change   (*Source*: Prochaska and DiClemente)

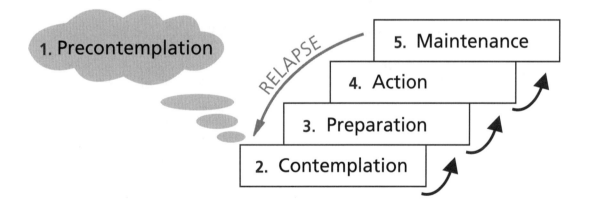

Stages of Change

STAGE 1   PRECONTEMPLATION: *Never; not yet ready to make change.*

- Uninterested in changing behavior
- Unaware of problem or risk

As far as I'm concerned, I don't have any problems that need changing.

STAGE 2   CONTEMPLATION: *Someday; thinking about making a change.*

- Aware that a problem exists
- Have considered change but feel stuck
- Have doubts about the long-term benefits of changing vs. the short-term inconvenience that change may bring

I know I need to exercise, but I just don't have the time right now.

I've been thinking about changing my eating habits, but I'm overwhelmed by all the conflicting nutrition information out there.

STAGE 3   PREPARATION: *Soon; making steps toward change.*

- Taking active steps to get ready to change
- Plan to take action within the next month
- May have unsuccessfully taken action in the past year

I am signed up to start a fitness class at the end of the month.

I have already decided that I want to change the way I eat.

STAGE 4   ACTION: *Now; on your way to healthy habits.*

- Practicing new behavior
- Realize that the action requires considerable time and energy

I'm working hard to be physically active on a regular basis.

I am making time for myself by placing my health needs high on my priority list.

STAGE 5   MAINTENANCE: *Ongoing; sustaining a healthy lifestyle.*

- Realize that new behavior is an important part of one's regular routine
- Consistently has ingrained the new behavior over the past six months

Exercise has become part of my lifestyle; I miss it when I skip a few days.

Eating a fruit and/or vegetable with every meal is automatic for me; I don't even have to think about it.

Navigating through Behavior Change

- You will find yourself in different stages for different health behaviors. For example, you may find it easy to shift to eating lower-fat foods (ACTION stage), but you may only be thinking about how to be more active during the week (CONTEMPLATION stage).

- You will move back and forth between stages. For example, you may be exercising regularly (ACTION stage) until you go on vacation. While on vacation, you stop exercising. Once you return home, you pick up a fitness class schedule so you can restart your fitness program (PREPARATION stage).

- You will find it easier to move from one stage to the next when you have realistic expectations and you don't judge yourself. If you fear imperfection, for example, you can be stuck in the CONTEMPLATION stage for years.

Are You Ready for Change Right Now?

Choosing to change or not to change is a personal decision. Making a major change always requires commitment and hard work, so you may want to consider whether this is the right time for you to be attempting significant lifestyle changes. Get started by spending ten to fifteen minutes to read and answer the following questions.

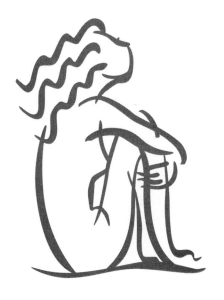

Is this a good time for change?

Consider your current time commitments, relationships, job status, health (yours and other family members') and financial status. Trying to change too many things at once sets you up to fail. For example, attempting to tackle your weight problem and stop smoking at the same time spells disaster. Likewise, your best intentions to lose or maintain a healthy weight will probably fall to the bottom of your priority list if you're in the middle of a personal crisis.

Is achieving a healthier weight worth the effort?

Change involves trade-offs such as giving up time in one area in order to devote time to a new, healthier behavior. Are you willing to make the trade-offs needed to meet your goal? For example, making more time for physical activity may mean less time reading or watching TV.

Only you know the personal costs and benefits of achieving a healthier weight. Take a few minutes and fill in the chart below to paint the whole picture before you decide.

Example:

Advantages of Changing	Disadvantages of Changing
• More energy	• Hard work/time-consuming
• Better health	• Difficult to find time for exercise
• Feel better about yourself	• Prefer foods high in fat
• Move easier	• Family prefers high-fat foods

Your list:

Advantages of Changing	Disadvantages of Changing
•	•
•	•
•	•
•	•

How committed are you to making changes?

You probably lead a busy life, so taking care of yourself and your needs won't happen unless you give them a prominent place on your list of things to do. To be successful at making lifestyle changes, you must be willing to place your personal goals at the top of your priority list. This means re-prioritizing your schedule and letting go of commitments that fall lower on your list.

Assessing Your Commitment Level

Most people who have lost weight and kept it off share the following characteristics: they exercise regularly; they eat less fat and fewer calories; and they build supportive relationships.

On a scale of 1 to 10, circle the number that best reflects your commitment to making physical activity part of your weekly routine.

0   1   2   3   4   5   6   7   8   9   (10)

Not Now   Ready and
                                                                               Committed

On a scale of 1 to 10, circle the number that best reflects your commitment to eating less fat and making nutritious food choices.

0   1   2   3   4   5   6   7   8   9   (10)

Not Now   Ready and
                                                                               Committed

On a scale of 1 to 10, circle the number that best reflects your commitment to support yourself by asking for help when you need it, being positive with the way you talk to yourself, and paying attention to your feelings and emotions.

0   1   2   3   4   5   6   7   8   9   (10)

Not Now   Ready and
                                                                               Committed

Is this the right time?

If you selected numbers between 0 and 3 on these scales . . .

You're not prepared to make major changes at this time. Think about what's happening in your life. Is it realistic to make any changes at this time? If you decide to continue with this program, be aware of your level of commitment and adjust your expectations accordingly. If you decide not to continue with this program, acknowledge and respect that you've made the right decision at this time. No time limit exists for changing behaviors. Next month or even next year may be a more reasonable time for change. When you're ready, be confident that you'll be able to make the changes needed to reach your goal.

If you selected numbers between 4 and 6 on these scales . . .

When it comes to making changes, you could land on either side of the fence. You want to change, but you may not be totally committed. You are most likely in either the CONTEMPLATION stage or PREPARATION stage of change. This program may or may not move you into the ACTION stage, but you can still benefit from making some smaller changes. Believing in yourself is one of the best predictors of success. How confident are you in your ability to make changes? If you think you can, you'll probably be successful with your efforts. If you think you will fail, you probably will.

If you selected numbers between 7 and 10 on these scales . . .

Now is a good time for you to make changes. You've selected the right program at the right time — congratulations! Making lifestyle changes is tough work. With the proper commitment and support, you can do it. The *Smart CHOICES* program will help you. With the tools and skills that you gain from this program and the support you receive from others, you can achieve your goals.

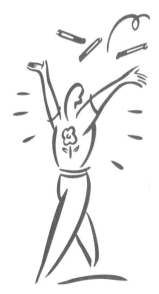

In the following weeks, you'll decide what to change and when to do it. You're in charge. Don't expect clear sailing. You'll undoubtedly encounter some rough waters on your journey toward better health. Move at your own pace. Slow down during stormy times and sail ahead when clear skies beckon.

Facts of Life: Measuring Your Progress

 Good health is defined by more than a number on a bathroom scale. It's about feeling good and having enough energy to do the things you want to do.

When it comes to making healthful lifestyle changes, you can measure your progress in many ways beyond just weighing yourself on a scale. Listed below are just a few. Take a couple of minutes and check off the behaviors and habits you want to work on in the upcoming weeks. Feel free to add some of your own. Monitor your progress by focusing on these areas along with watching your weight.

Short- and Long-Term Indicators of Progress:

Some of these changes can take place right away (a few days to a few weeks); others will take longer.

Healthier Eating Habits:

☒ Eat more fruits and vegetables.

☒ Eat more complex carbohydrates, such as whole grains and dried beans (legumes).

☒ Make lower-fat food choices.

☒ Plan ahead more often regarding meals and snacks.

☒ Eat smaller amounts.

Better Emotional Health:

☒ Pay more attention to my body's hunger/fullness signals (eat when hungry, stop before feeling stuffed).

☐ Do less dieting; give up trying to rigidly control what I eat.

☐ Improve my attitude toward my body (stop negative self-talk).

☒ Feel more at peace with food and the role it plays in my life.

☐ Be less critical of myself (less negative self-talk).

☒ Feel more capable of achieving and maintaining a healthier weight.

☐ Do less emotional eating or bingeing (use food less often as a coping mechanism).

☒ Ask for support more often.

☒ Be more assertive in turning down food when not hungry.

Improved Physical Health:

- ☐ Move with greater ease.
- ☐ Lose body fat (forget the scale; measure inches lost with a tape measure).
- ☒ Feel less short of breath when climbing stairs or carrying packages.
- ☒ Feel more comfortable in my clothes.
- ☐ Be able to participate more fully in fun physical activities (such as hiking with the family).
- ☐ Have more energy throughout the day (fewer highs and lows).
- ☐ Be more physically active on a consistent, regular basis.

Improved Medical Status:

- ☐ Improve diabetes control.
- ☐ Lower my blood pressure.
- ☐ Lower my cholesterol level.
- ☐ Be able to take less medication for a chronic health problem or illness.
- ☐ Other Changes: _____

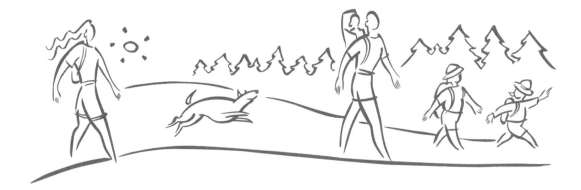

Using a Tape Measure to Track Progress

 Jumping on and off the scale gives you a number, but it doesn't provide a very clear picture of what's happening to your body. What does the number on the scale represent? Are you losing muscle, fat or water?

To find out the truth, set aside your scale and take out a tape measure. To track changes in body fat, simply take your measurements and track them over time. Inches lost represent a decrease in body fat, even though the number on the scale may not budge.

Most people resist taking their measurements. You'll be glad you did when you witness the changes that can take place in a few short weeks. Don't worry about the exact numbers. What matters is watching these numbers change over time. Grab a tape measure and get started.

Steps for Taking Measurements:

1. With a pliable tape measure in hand, find a full-length mirror so you can watch yourself while you measure each area. As you measure, turn sideways and make sure the tape measure is straight across, front to back. For the most accurate measurements, wear minimal clothing.

2. Measure your chest/bust, hips, arms and thighs at their fullest part; measure your waist at its narrowest part. You can measure above or below your belly button, just be consistent and re-measure the same area every time. To detect changes, select the areas of your body that carry the most fat.

3. When taking measurements of your bust/chest, waist and hips, keep your posture straight. Pull the measuring tape tight but not so snug that you indent the skin.

4. Take two measurements of each body part. Measure to the nearest 1/4 inch. If your two measurements aren't the same, take a third one and record the average.

5. Each time you re-measure in subsequent weeks, measure at the same spot.

6. Make notes about the exact location you measure. Use moles, birthmarks or a set number of inches from a joint as landmarks. For example, if you are measuring your thigh, measure xxx number of inches up your leg from the top of your kneecap. Mark this spot with a pen. Take your measurement at that spot.

Body Measurements

	NOTES	WEEK 1	WEEK 5	WEEK 10
Date		9 - 21		
Bust/chest		35½		
Waist/stomach		23 w 36 st.		
Hips		43		
Right thigh		24		
Right upper arm		12½		

The Fitness Solution

 When it comes to losing weight and keeping it off, the "movers and shakers" always come out ahead. Sure, you need to select nutritious foods, but if you don't move, you're not going to lose. Getting started may be tough, but the rewards will keep you going.

Why Be Active?

If a magic pill existed that could help you lose weight, live longer, handle stress better, and reduce your risk of heart disease, cancer and diabetes — without any side effects — would you take it? This may sound too good to be true, but an active lifestyle provides all of these health benefits and more. Dust off your sneakers and get moving:

- Control your weight and reduce your body fat.

- Increase your metabolism. Your body burns calories during exercise and even after you stop.

- Increase your muscle mass, which in turn will increase your metabolism.

- Reduce your health risks — physical activity lowers your risk for heart disease, stroke, high blood pressure, diabetes, osteoporosis and certain types of cancer. It can also reduce the progression of arthritis.

- Improve your endurance and stamina; feel less tired.

- Sleep better.

- Feel less tense and anxious; handle stress better.

- Strengthen your muscles, bones and ligaments.

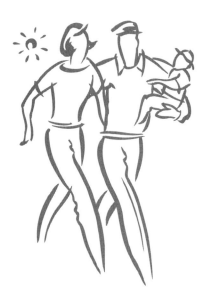

The benefits you gain depend on how often and how long you exercise, as well as what activity you choose to do. For example, a walk around the block may help you sleep better, but it won't burn off the double helpings you ate at dinner. Do you need to join a health club to get these benefits? Not necessarily, but a good pair of walking shoes can help. Anytime you physically move or exercise, you burn calories. The bottom line — move more as often as you can.

Before You Start a Fitness Program

Check with your doctor before you start exercising. Don't ignore this advice — especially if you have certain medical conditions (such as high blood pressure, high cholesterol, or a personal or family history of heart disease), are pregnant, smoke cigarettes, or are over age 40 (for men) or over age 50 (for women). You shouldn't have any problems if you start out slow and gradually build up to more strenuous activities. For more specific guidelines, seek help from a qualified fitness professional.

What to Expect When You Start a Fitness Program

Expect some stiffness or soreness when you first start a new activity, but NOT pain. Sore muscles let you know that your exercise program is working! Muscle soreness usually disappears in a few days. On the other hand, pain is a signal that something is wrong. If you experience pain or feel yourself getting overtired or out of breath during exercise, check with your doctor or a fitness professional.

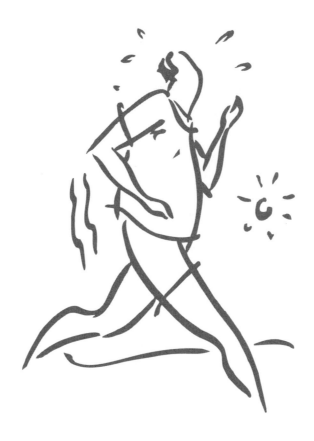

Exploring Your Fitness Options

Have you ever started an exercise program, only to have it fizzle from boredom after a few weeks? Go for activities you enjoy so you can stick with your fitness plan. Take a few minutes to explore what these activities may be for you.

What activities do you enjoy that fit into your schedule? As you explore your options, take five minutes to write down your answers to the following questions.

- What fitness activities do I enjoy (e.g., recreational sports, vigorous yardwork/ gardening, walking, etc.)?

- Do I prefer being inside or outside?

- Do I mind sweating or do I prefer less strenuous activities?

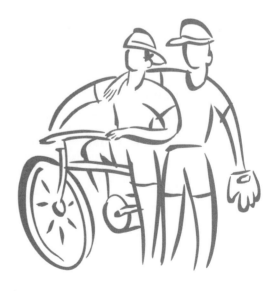

- Do I enjoy exercising alone (swimming, walking, stationary bike) or would I prefer to exercise with a group (aerobic or swing dancing, group cycling/ walking/running)?

List your favorite way(s) to stay active:

Ideas: walking, swimming, aerobic fitness class, cycling, swing dancing, hiking

This week, what steps will you take to move forward with these activities?

I intend to . . . (Check all that apply):

☐ Get medical consent from my physician.

☐ Call for or pick up a swimming pool schedule or fitness class schedule.

☐ Purchase a new pair of walking shoes.

☐ Arrange for child care.

☐ Enlist a fitness partner.

☐ Rent or borrow a piece of fitness equipment for a trial test before purchasing.

☐ Get information about joining a club.

☐ Go through my closet and pull out comfortable clothes for exercise.

☐ Other: _____

Keeping Track: Food & Activity Journal

 A habit refers to a behavior that has been repeated so often it becomes automatic. In order to change a habit, be it smoking, drinking or eating, you need to first understand the behaviors entangled in the habit. Play Sherlock Holmes and observe your current eating behaviors. You can't consciously change what you're not aware of. As you gather clues and evidence over the next ten weeks, you will unveil some of the mystery that stands between you and a healthier lifestyle.

Step One: Gathering clues

Using the FOOD & ACTIVITY JOURNAL at the end of this chapter, write down everything that you crunch on, slurp up and slip into your mouth for one week. Try NOT to make any changes in the way you eat this week. As much as possible, simply observe and record your eating patterns without making any changes or judgments.

Step Two: Making every bit of evidence count

Don't forget to record snacks and beverages. Write down everything, including the handful of peanuts you grab at your meeting and the "taste tests" you take while preparing dinner. Start to keep a record first thing tomorrow morning. Your JOURNAL also contains a place to record your physical activity (in minutes or miles). Now turn to page 21 and review the guidelines on HOW TO KEEP A FOOD & ACTIVITY JOURNAL.

> How will you remember to write in your FOOD & ACTIVITY JOURNAL? Where will you keep your JOURNAL so you won't forget about it? These ideas should help you stay on track.
>
> Keep your JOURNAL within easy reach:
> - In your day planner
> - On your kitchen or dining room table
> - On your desk
>
> Use cues to help yourself remember:
> - Leave Post-it Notes to yourself everywhere — on the bathroom mirror, in your car, on your day planner, by your bed.
> - Write it on your calendar at home and at work.
> - Ask a supportive friend or family member to remind you. Be specific about how you would like them to remind you. What would you like them to say? When should they remind you? How often should they remind you?

Step Three: Solving the mystery

You probably won't solve the entire mystery after just one week of recording clues and evidence in your FOOD & ACTIVITY JOURNAL. But you will have a much clearer picture of what's happening with your eating habits. At the end of the week, you'll be ready to reflect on the information you've gathered and make some decisions based on what you found.

Facts of Life: Food for Thought

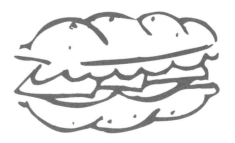

Studies show a connection between record keeping and success with losing weight and keeping it off. So use your FOOD & ACTIVITY JOURNAL to monitor your eating habits. It's easiest to start by tracking the foods you eat. Later on, you can look at hunger/fullness cues, calories, fat and emotional aspects of eating. With each passing week, you gain more and more insight into why you eat the way you do. Consider the different options for monitoring eating habits that are listed each week under the Skill Practice section. Choose the one that best meets your needs.

Your daily routine probably doesn't include writing down everything that you eat, so it may seem difficult to do at first. To keep an accurate FOOD & ACTIVITY JOURNAL requires time and effort on your part. Like any new behavior, it becomes easier with practice. Do the work now and reap the benefits for a lifetime.

Some people feel as if they are on a diet when they keep food records. If you feel this way — STOP! Food records should help you become more aware of your habits and help you monitor your progress. Food records should not bring out the "food police" or "closet dieter" in you. Remind yourself that diets don't work. Your goal is to learn more about yourself and your eating habits. There is no "right" or "wrong" way to eat, no "good" or "bad" foods. Fill out those portions of the FOOD & ACTIVITY JOURNAL that you feel comfortable with.

How to Keep a FOOD & ACTIVITY JOURNAL

You'll find a FOOD & ACTIVITY JOURNAL located at the end of each chapter. Feel free to make photocopies if you want or need extra pages. Start with a new page each day. Write in each journal as soon as possible after eating a meal or snack.

Use your FOOD & ACTIVITY JOURNAL each week to track a different aspect of your eating habits. Aim to record in your journal for a minimum of three days (two weekdays and one weekend day). If you find this activity useful, continue for the entire week.

Fill in the unshaded columns of each journal. In Week One, for example, you'll complete only the Fitness Activity, Time, Food and Drink, and Amounts sections of the journal.

Fitness Activity	Record the type of activity and the number of minutes or miles (in the space next to "Fitness Activity"). *Do not include daily household chores.*
Time	Record the time whenever you eat or drink something other than water (e.g., 5:00 p.m.).
Feelings Check	In Week Six, check in with your mood or feelings before eating and record your observations (e.g., content, frustrated, angry, tired, bored, depressed, rushed, etc.).
Hunger/Fullness Scale (Range: 0–10)	In Week Two, rate your degree of hunger before each meal/snack and how full you feel after each meal/snack.
Food & Drink	Write down everything you eat or drink throughout the day including snacks, coffee, and alcoholic or non-alcoholic beverages. BE SPECIFIC. If you ate a turkey sandwich, for example, list: two slices sourdough bread, three ounces turkey, one tablespoon light mayonnaise.
Amounts	Use household measurements to indicate amounts (e.g., cups, tablespoons, teaspoons). Measure meat and cheese in ounces.
Calories	In Week Three, track your calories to see how you spend them. Obtain calorie information from the Nutrition Facts section of food labels and the CALORIE & FAT COUNTER (pages 255-280). Total your calories each day.
Fat	In Week Four, record the foods you eat and the amount of fat they contain (in grams). Obtain information on fat (grams) from the Nutrition Facts section of food labels and the CALORIE & FAT COUNTER (pages 255-280). Total your fat grams each day.

Skill Practice: Week One

 It's important to recognize the difference between "skill power" and willpower. For you to make lifestyle changes, skill power will serve you better than plain old willpower. Willpower implies that you must deprive yourself or hold yourself back. Many people believe they simply weren't born with this ability. On the contrary, you can learn new behaviors or skills at any time. Having the right skills in place will empower you to make positive lifestyle changes. To brush up on your skill power, spend some time on these activities in the upcoming week.

1. **Keep records** — Write down everything that you eat and drink in your FOOD & ACTIVITY JOURNAL. Try NOT to change your eating habits this week. Simply observe your current patterns.

2. **Follow through on EXPLORING YOUR FITNESS OPTIONS** — Complete this activity if you haven't already done so, then follow through on the items you checked off. Taking these steps moves you closer to an active lifestyle. Record any exercise or fitness activities you do this week in your FOOD & ACTIVITY JOURNAL in the space provided.

3. **Take your body measurements** — Set aside your scale and grab a tape measure. Fill in the numbers on the chart on page 14. These numbers will serve as a starting point against which you can compare future measurements.

Reminder: Don't forget to record your fitness activities in your FOOD & ACTIVITY JOURNAL.

FOOD & ACTIVITY JOURNAL

Date:_____

Day: M   Tu   W   Th   F   Sat   Sun

Fitness Activity:

TIME	FEELINGS CHECK	H/F SCALE*	FOOD & DRINK	AMOUNT	CALORIES	FAT (grams)	H/F SCALE*
7:00 a.m.			Poppyseed bagel	1 large			
			Cream cheese, Regular	2 Tbsp.			
			1% Milk	8 oz.			
			OJ	6 oz.			
			Coffee	2 cups			
11:30 a.m.			Turkey sandwich:				
			Whole wheat bread	2 slices			
			Turkey breast	3 oz.			
			Light mayo	1 Tbsp.			
			Lettuce	1 piece			
			Baked low-fat chips	2 oz.			
			Apple	1			
			1% Milk	8 oz.			
3:30 p.m.			Bag of pretzels	2.5 oz.			
			Diet soda	12 oz.			
6:30 p.m.			Spaghetti:				
			Pasta	1 1/2 cups			
			Tomato sauce with meat	1/2 cup			
			French bread	2 slices			
			Margarine	2 tsp.			
			Tossed salad	2 cups			
			Low-fat Italian dressing	2 Tbsp.			
			Red wine	6 oz.			
9:00 p.m.			Bowl lite ice cream	1 cup			
					Total:	Total:	

*Rate your hunger/fullness on a scale from 0–10: 0 = Empty, 5 = Just Right, 10 = Stuffed

FOOD & ACTIVITY JOURNAL

Date: Thurs - 21

Day: M Tu W Th F Sat Sun

Fitness Activity:

TIME	FEELINGS CHECK	H/F SCALE*	FOOD & DRINK	AMOUNT	CALORIES	FAT (grams)	H/F SCALE*
7:30			cereal	1 cup			
			milk	1/2 cup			
			coffee	1 cup			
			creamer	2 TBL			
10:15			chicken nuggets	8			
			chips Tortilla w/cheese	10			
			Berries mixed	1/2 c.			
			Peaches	3 slices			
			water	6 oz			
4:30			Bean + Beef Burrito	1			
			lettuce	1/2 c			
			milk	5 oz			
					Total:	Total:	

*Rate your hunger/fullness on a scale from 0–10: 0 = Empty, 5 = Just Right, 10 = Stuffed

FOOD & ACTIVITY JOURNAL

Date: _Fri 22_

Day: M   Tu   W   Th   F   Sat   Sun

Fitness Activity:

TIME	FEELINGS CHECK	H/F SCALE*	FOOD & DRINK	AMOUNT	CALORIES	FAT (grams)	H/F SCALE*
7:30			Toast (whole wheat oat)	2 pieces			
			Butter	1 tsp			
			cereal	1 c			
			milk	1/2 c.			
10:20			Fruit mixed	1 cup			
			water	4 oz			
5:00			chicken	3 small pieces			
			Green Beans	1/2 c			
			Tomatoe sliced	1 medium			
			milk	6 oz.			
					Total:	Total:	

*Rate your hunger/fullness on a scale from 0–10: 0 = Empty, 5 = Just Right, 10 = Stuffed

FOOD & ACTIVITY JOURNAL

Date: Sat 23

Day: M Tu W Th F Sat Sun

Fitness Activity:

TIME	FEELINGS CHECK	H/F SCALE*	FOOD & DRINK	AMOUNT	CALORIES	FAT (grams)	H/F SCALE*
9:00			Banana Bread orange juice	2 slices 4 oz			
12:00			chicken noodle soup Juice	1½ c. 4 oz			
5:00			Beef Stroganoff Rice Green Beans tomato slices cucumber Apple Pie ice cream milk	1½ c. 1 c ½ c 3 5 slices 1 small piece 2 scoops 6 oz			
					Total:	Total:	

*Rate your hunger/fullness on a scale from 0–10: 0 = Empty, 5 = Just Right, 10 = Stuffed

FOOD & ACTIVITY JOURNAL

Date: Sun 24

Day: M Tu W Th F Sat Sun

Fitness Activity:

TIME	FEELINGS CHECK	H/F SCALE*	FOOD & DRINK	AMOUNT	CALORIES	FAT (grams)	H/F SCALE*
9:30			Cereal	1 c			
			milk	1/2 c			
			Banana Bread	1 slice			
			Butter	1/2 ts			
12:30			coffee ice cream	2 scoops			
5:00			Halibut				
			Salad mixed	1 1/2 c			
			oel + ven. dressing	TBL			
			tomatoes	2 slices			
			olives	1 TBL			
			sunflower seed	1 TBL			
			Red Potatoe's	2-1 cup			
					Total:	Total:	

*Rate your hunger/fullness on a scale from 0–10: 0 = Empty, 5 = Just Right, 10 = Stuffed

FOOD & ACTIVITY JOURNAL

Date: mon 25

Day: M Tu W Th F Sat Sun

Fitness Activity:

TIME	FEELINGS CHECK	H/F SCALE*	FOOD & DRINK	AMOUNT	CALORIES	FAT (grams)	H/F SCALE*
7:30			cereal	1 cup			
			milk	1/2 c			
10:30			Salad	1 cup			
			Beets	2 slices			
			mushroom	1			
			ceasar dress.	2 TBL			
			Sunflower seeds	1 TBL			
			1 carton choc milk	small			
			spanish Rice	1/4 c			
5:30			Turkey + Ham Sandwich	3 g			
			Bread	2 slices			
			milkshake	8 g			
					Total:	Total:	

*Rate your hunger/fullness on a scale from 0–10: 0 = Empty, 5 = Just Right, 10 = Stuffed

FOOD & ACTIVITY JOURNAL

Date: Tues 26

Day: M **Tu** W Th F Sat Sun

Fitness Activity:

TIME	FEELINGS CHECK	H/F SCALE*	FOOD & DRINK	AMOUNT	CALORIES	FAT (grams)	H/F SCALE*
7.30			cereal	1 cup			
			milk	1/2 c			
10.15			salad	1 c			
			mushroom	1			
			pears	2 pieces			
			water	4 g			
			milk	small c.			
5.30			orange juice	4 oz			
			Brocolli cass.	1 1/2 cup			
			Brocolli	1 cup			
			cheese cheddar	1/4 c			
			mushroom soup				
			Rolls	2			
			Butter	1 TB		Total:	
			choc cake				
			milk	4 oz e			

*Rate your hunger/fullness on a scale from 0–10: 0 = Empty, 5 = Just Right, 10 = Stuffed

FOOD & ACTIVITY JOURNAL

Date: Wed 27

Day: M Tu W Th F Sat Sun

Fitness Activity:

TIME	FEELINGS CHECK	H/F SCALE*	FOOD & DRINK	AMOUNT	CALORIES	FAT (grams)	H/F SCALE*
7:30			cereal milk	1 c 1/2			
10:15			salad mix Berries mix	1/2 c 1/4 c			
2:00			Hamburger cheese lettuce Salad water Beer Dressing	 1 slice 1 leaf 8 oz 8 oz 1 tbl.			
					Total:	Total:	

*Rate your hunger/fullness on a scale from 0–10: 0 = Empty, 5 = Just Right, 10 = Stuffed

Dig In and Move Out

Welcome back! Every time you delve into this workbook, you strengthen your commitment toward reaching a healthier weight and enjoying a more healthful lifestyle.

> ## This Week You Will:
>
> - Reflect over the previous week, noting insights and accomplishments.
> - Learn how to make healthier food choices using the Food Guide Pyramid.
> - Recognize the value of building meals around complex carbohydrates.
> - Tune into your body's hunger and fullness signals when eating.
> - Learn how to make time for physical activity.
> - Design a personal S.M.A.R.T. plan for fitness.

Reflections

 Take a few minutes and look at the FOOD & ACTIVITY JOURNAL you kept this past week. Keeping in mind the stages of change (never, someday, soon, now), ask yourself what behaviors and habits you are ready to change. For example, you may be willing to work on fitting in a daily walk, but you can't even think about giving up ice cream as a bedtime snack.

What behaviors and habits are you ready and willing to change now? What areas of your lifestyle are you NOT willing to change at this point in time? Jot down your thoughts below.

Ready and Willing to Change Now	Not Willing to Change at This Time

Take another moment and think about the EXPLORING YOUR FITNESS OPTIONS checklist from last week. What steps did you take that will help you become more active in the weeks ahead?

If you didn't keep a FOOD & ACTIVITY JOURNAL last week

Stop now and catch yourself before you slip too far off-track. Take a few minutes and ask yourself why you didn't record in your journal. What got in your way? Write your answer(s) below.

Example: Kept forgetting to write down what I ate during the day.

It can be tedious keeping records; however, it's a vital part of changing habits. When you take the time to write everything down, it helps you focus on and stay committed to your long-term goal of becoming a healthier person. Take a minute and write down some suggestions that would help you accomplish your record keeping in the upcoming week.

What I will do differently:

Example: I will stick an index card in my day planner each day to record on. At night I will copy what
I ate into my workbook.

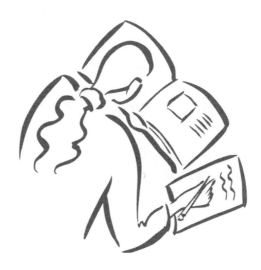

The Food Guide Pyramid: Eating Right Made Easy

 Need some help choosing healthier foods? Check out the Food Guide Pyramid. It organizes foods into categories according to the nutrients they provide. Generous amounts of plant-based foods such as breads, cereals and grains (complex carbohydrates), and fruits and vegetables form the foundation of the pyramid. You'll find moderate amounts of meat (and meat alternates) and dairy foods on the next level. Finally, the tip of the pyramid contains a sprinkling of foods that are high in sugar and/or fat and low in other nutrients.

Each food group contributes specific nutrients to your diet. The foods in one group cannot replace foods in another. That's why eating a variety of foods is so important. Besides, variety is the spice of life! Stop for a moment and take a closer look at this guide to optimal nutrition.

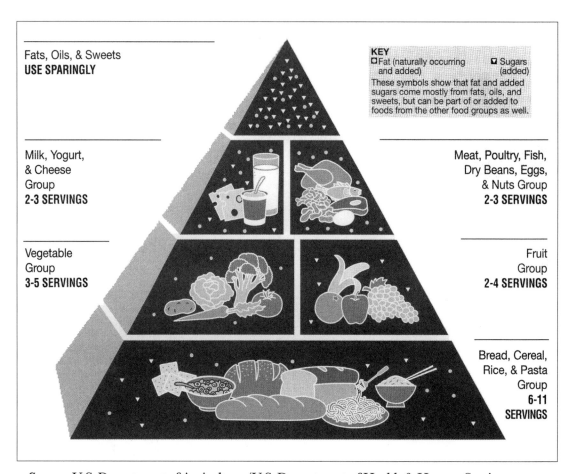

Source: U.S. Department of Agriculture/U.S. Department of Health & Human Services

Bread, Cereal, Rice and Pasta Group — 6–11 Servings

Serving sizes: 1 slice of bread; 1 tortilla; 1/2 cup rice, pasta or cooked cereal; 1 ounce of cold cereal; 1/2 of a hamburger roll, bagel (small) or English muffin; 3-4 plain crackers; 1 pancake (4-inch).

Found at the base of the Pyramid, grains and starches provide complex carbohydrates, B vitamins and fiber. At first glance, the six to 11 servings might seem like a lot. In fact, the serving sizes are fairly small and add up quickly. For example, many people typically eat two cups (or four servings) of pasta at one meal.

For a fiber boost, choose whole grain foods such as whole wheat bread, whole grain crackers, brown rice and other grains.

Vegetable and Fruit Groups — 5+ Servings

Serving sizes: 1/2 cup raw, cooked or canned; 1 cup raw, leafy vegetables; 3/4 cup (6 oz.) juice; 1/4 cup dried fruit; 1 medium fresh fruit.

Don't pass up a nutritional bargain! Fruits and vegetables are low in calories and loaded with carbohydrates, vitamins A and C, fiber, and health-protective phytochemicals (active plant compounds that protect against heart disease and cancer).

If you get confused about the recommended minimum number of daily servings, think "five a day." Choose dark, colorful fruits and vegetables, such as spinach, cantaloupe and sweet potatoes, which pack more nutritional value than pale iceberg lettuce or celery.

Meat, Poultry, Fish, Dry Beans, Eggs and Nuts Group — 2–3 Servings

Serving sizes: 2–3 ounces cooked meat, poultry or fish. Each of the following is equivalent to 1 ounce of meat: 1/2 cup cooked beans or tofu, 1 egg, 2 tablespoons peanut butter, 1/3 cup nuts.

These protein-rich foods supply important nutrients such as B vitamins, iron and zinc. To cut down on artery-clogging saturated fat and cholesterol, choose lean cuts of meat, poultry without skin, fish, and dried beans and peas (such as lentils, split peas and kidney beans).

Stretch your fat budget, and your pocketbook, by keeping an eye on your portions. Three ounces of cooked lean meat, poultry or fish is about the size of a deck of cards. Go easy on high-fat items such as nuts and seeds.

For a nutrition bonus, eat dishes with dried beans, lentils and peas. These foods provide protein and fiber without the fat. They're also an excellent source of complex carbohydrates and could be in the base of the pyramid with the grains.

Milk, Yogurt and Cheese Group — 2–3 Servings

Children and teens (9-18 years) and older adults (51+ years) need 4 servings.

Serving sizes: 1 cup (8 oz.) milk or yogurt, 1 1/2 – 2 ounces cheese, 1 1/2 cup ice cream, 1 cup frozen yogurt. Each serving provides approximately 300 milligrams of calcium.

Select low-fat varieties of dairy foods to fill up on protein, calcium and vitamin D. Dairy products are nature's best source of calcium, a mineral that builds strong bones and prevents osteoporosis. For sources of calcium, refer to the chart on the next page.

Fats, Oils and Sweets — Limit or Use Sparingly

The tip of the Pyramid contains foods that supply calories, fat and sugar, but little else in the way of good nutrition. Nevertheless, don't think of these foods as "bad" — a healthy diet has room for small amounts. Go easy on fats and sugars you add to foods in cooking or at the table: butter, margarine, oil, cream, gravy, salad dressing, sugar and jelly. Choose fewer foods that are high in sugar: soft drinks, candy, cookies and other sweet desserts.

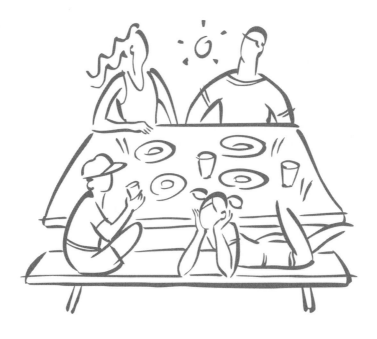

Calcium Sources

Adult Calcium Needs: 1000–1200 mgs a day *

CALCIUM (milligrams)	FOOD	SERVING SIZE
300 – 350 mgs	Yogurt, low-fat	1 cup
	Milk (nonfat, low-fat, lactose reduced, whole, chocolate, buttermilk)	1 cup
	Calcium-fortified orange juice	1 cup
200 – 250 mgs	Cheese, most hard varieties	1 ounce
	Ice cream/frozen yogurt, low-fat	1 cup
	Ricotta cheese, low-fat	1/4 cup
	Total cereal	3/4 cup
150 – 200 mgs	Collard greens, cooked	1/2 cup
	Instant oatmeal	1 packet
	Puddings, flan, custards	1/2 cup
	Salmon, canned, with bones	3 ounces
100 – 150 mgs	Sardines, canned, drained	1 ounce
	Tofu (made with calcium sulfate)	3 ounces
50 – 100 mgs	Almonds, shelled	1 ounce
	Beans, most dried varieties	1/2 cup
	Beet greens, kale, bok choy	1/2 cup
	Cottage cheese, low-fat	1/2 cup
	Orange	1 medium
	Parmesan cheese, grated	1 Tbsp
	Calcium-fortified soy milk and rice milk	1 cup
25 – 50 mgs	Bread	2 slices
	Broccoli, cooked	1/2 cup
	Corn tortilla	1 medium

*1997 Dietary Reference Intakes (new RDAs), Institute of Medicine, National Academy of Sciences

Note: The calcium content of products may vary from brand to brand.

Supplements

If you don't think you get all the calcium you need from food, consider taking a calcium carbonate or calcium citrate supplement. Avoid supplements containing bone meal, oyster shell or dolomite due to possible metal contamination.

Power Up With Complex Carbohydrates

 Most of the calories in your diet should come from grain products, vegetables and fruit. Take another look at the Food Guide Pyramid. Grain products such as breads, cereals, pasta and rice form the foundation of a healthy diet. Rich in complex carbohydrates, these foods receive top marks from nutrition experts for the following reasons:

• Naturally low in fat, sugar and salt.

• Excellent source of vitamins (especially the B vitamins) and minerals.

• More filling for fewer calories than high-fat or high-sugar foods.

• Inexpensive, easy to prepare and tasty.

• If high in fiber, promote regularity and help prevent constipation and hemorrhoids.

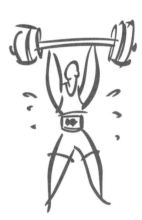

Eating healthy means building meals around complex carbohydrates (breads, pasta, rice, beans and potatoes), fruits and vegetables. Foods high in complex carbohydrates are not fattening. Blame the extra fat and calories on the cream cheese that tops your bagel or the Alfredo sauce you pour over pasta. The trick is to limit the *fat* that often accompanies high-carbohydrate foods: sour cream or butter on baked potatoes, cream or cheese sauces on pasta, and peanut butter on bread.

Building Meals around Complex Carbohydrates

In our culture, we traditionally emphasize meals planned around meat. To eat more complex carbohydrates, think of meat as a side dish, not the main attraction. Rely on meat as you would any other condiment — use it to flavor dishes. Here are a few examples of meals where meat takes the backseat: spaghetti with meatballs, shish kebabs with rice, stir-fry with noodles, chili, or soup with bread or crackers.

Building meals around complex carbohydrates takes some planning. The chart on the following page provides some examples to get you started. Add your own ideas to the list.

COMPLEX CARBOHYDRATE	MEAL IDEAS
POTATO	Baked potato topped with low-fat chili, low-fat cheese, low-fat cottage cheese or salsa; scalloped potatoes made with skim milk and a small amount of ham; beef stew (heavy on the vegetables and potatoes, light on the meat)
BEANS	Bean burritos, beans and rice, bean soups (black bean, lentil, minestrone, split pea)
RICE	Stir-fry, casseroles, soups, beans and rice, pilafs
BREAD	Soup and bread; sandwiches with low-fat spreads; pizza made from focaccia, pita or french bread (easy on the cheese)
PASTA	Minestrone soup; macaroni and cheese made without butter; pasta with a low-fat sauce: • Marinara sauce (add veggies, artichokes or beans) • Creamy basil (1 cup low-fat sour cream with 1 tablespoon of pesto) • Primavera sauce
TORTILLA	Chicken fajitas, bean burritos, and nachos made with low-fat ingredients

Tips

- Keep extra cooked rice or pasta in the refrigerator to reheat and eat.

- Stock the cupboard with ingredients for several "quickie" meals. Examples: for burritos, stock canned low-fat refried beans, tortillas and salsa; for pizza, stock frozen focaccia bread, shredded skim milk mozzarella cheese, and bottled spaghetti or marinara sauce.

- Always have good-quality bread on hand to round out a meal. Bread can easily be frozen; just double wrap to prevent freezer burn.

Boost Your Fiber

Why eat a fiber-rich diet?

- Fiber fills you up, so you tend to eat less.

- The fiber in food helps lower blood cholesterol and reduce heart disease.

- High-fiber foods move through your intestines, preventing constipation, and may help reduce the risk of colon cancer.

- Fiber-rich foods help keep blood sugar levels more stable.

How much fiber do you need?

The National Cancer Institute recommends eating 20-30 grams of fiber per day.

Good Sources of Fiber:

Cereals	Fiber (grams)
General Mills Fiber One, 1/2 cup	13
Wheat bran, 1/2 cup	13
Kellogg's All Bran, 1/2 cup	10
Post Fruit & Fibre, 1 cup	10
Wheatena, 1 cup	8
Kellogg's Raisin Bran, 1 cup	7
Ralston Chex 100% Whole Wheat, 1 cup	7
Quaker Oat Bran, cooked, 1 cup	6
Nabisco Spoon Size Shredded Wheat, 1 cup	5
Post Grape-Nuts, 1/2 cup	5
Oatmeal, cooked, 1 cup	4.5

Breads, Grains, Legumes, Pasta	Fiber (grams)
Barley, pearl, cooked, 1 cup	9
Black-eyed peas, canned, 1/2 cup	8.5
Black, pinto or kidney beans, 1/2 cup	8
Baked beans, 1/2 cup	7
Bulgur, cooked, 1 cup	7
Spaghetti, whole wheat, cooked, 1 cup	6
Refried beans, 1/2 cup	6
Lentils, 1/2 cup	4
Rice, brown, cooked, 1 cup	3.5
Bran muffin, 1 small	3
Bread, 100% whole wheat or whole grain, 1 slice	2

Fruits	Fiber (grams)
Blackberries and raspberries, fresh, 1 cup	8-9
Apple, unpeeled, 1 medium	5
Cranberries, dried, 1/2 cup	5
Figs, dried, 3	5
Grapefruit, 1/2 medium	5
Orange, 1 medium	5
Pear, with skin, 1 medium	5
Apricots, dried, 10	4
Prunes, dried, 5	4
Raisins, 1/2 cup	4
Strawberries, 1 cup	4

Vegetables	Fiber (grams)
Baked potato, with skin, 1 medium	4
Sweet potato, without skin, 1 medium	3.5
Brussels sprouts, cooked, 1/2 cup	3.5
Corn, cooked, 1/2 cup	3.5
Peas, cooked, 1/2 cup	3
Winter squash, cooked, 1/2 cup	3
Carrot, 1 medium	2.5
Broccoli, cooked, 1/2 cup	2
Spinach, cooked, 1/2 cup	2

Snacks	Fiber (grams)
Popcorn, 3 cups	4

Note: The fiber content of products may vary from brand to brand.

Caution! Adjust to a higher-fiber diet by *gradually* increasing your fiber intake and by drinking lots of water.

Facts of Life: Tuning in to Physical Hunger

Eating should be a pleasurable, guilt-free experience. Unfortunately, this isn't always true, especially if you've been riding the dieting roller coaster. Diets tend to moralize food, placing it into "good" and "bad" categories. Judgments about food as well as the dieting mentality can disconnect you from your body's internal feelings of hunger and fullness. Instead of relying on these internal cues to regulate when, what and how much to eat, you allow external triggers (sight or smell of food, diets, emotions) to dictate your body's need for food.

Is Your Head Ruling Your Stomach?

When you reach for food because you experience physical hunger, you are listening to your body's internal cues. You are less likely to overeat if you listen and respond to internal cues (hunger and fullness) rather than external cues (sight or smell of food, emotions). Having a healthy relationship with food goes beyond eating carrots and beans. It means:

- Choosing when to eat by paying attention to internal signals of hunger.

- Deciding how much food to eat by listening to fullness signals.

- Recognizing when you turn to food for emotional reasons.

The first step is to become more aware of hunger and fullness signals. Take a moment and think about what it means to be truly hungry. What does hunger feel like for you? Do you ever let yourself get hungry?

Check all the boxes below that apply:

❑ My stomach growls.

❑ I feel weak, dizzy or light-headed.

❑ I sometimes get a headache.

❑ Other: _____

❑ I don't know, I never let myself get hungry.

Working with a Hunger/Fullness Scale

Sometimes you may find it difficult to know why you need to eat. Are you physically hungry or are you eating for some other reason? The HUNGER/FULLNESS SCALE can help you make this distinction. This valuable tool helps you separate physical hunger from emotional hunger or other environmental cues that can lead to overeating.

HUNGER   FULLNESS

0 ....5 10

Starved   Comfortable   Stuffed

   0 = You feel starved or ravenous. You haven't eaten anything in many hours.

   5 = You feel comfortable and satisfied, neither hungry nor full.

 10 = You feel stuffed (like after Thanksgiving dinner).

The HUNGER/FULLNESS SCALE gives you immediate feedback regarding the *internal* state of your body. See if you can identify with or tap into your physical needs at these points on the scale.

Getting too hungry . . .

If you reach "0" or "1" on the scale, you've allowed yourself to get too hungry. Your best intentions to eat healthy foods fly out the window at this point. You settle for eating anything you can get your hands on. Getting too hungry sets you up for overeating. You devour foods quickly, not even tasting or enjoying them, and you're more likely to miss the "I'm full" signal when your body sends it.

Just right . . .

When you reach "5" on the scale, you feel satisfied and comfortable — neither hungry nor full.

Becoming too full . . .

If you eat to a "10" on the scale, you've overdone it. You want to eat until you feel *satisfied*, not to the point of feeling *full* or *stuffed*. At a "10," you've stopped listening to your body's internal cues and you are eating in response to environmental cues or emotional hunger.

Practice Helps

In the upcoming week, practice using the HUNGER/FULLNESS SCALE. It will help you tune in to your physical hunger and recognize when you overeat for other reasons. Don't get hung up on the numbers; everyone's scale will be slightly different. Take a few seconds to check in with your body's hunger/fullness signals before, while and after you eat. The following questions will help guide you in this process.

Before you put something into your mouth, ask yourself:

- Where am I on the HUNGER/FULLNESS SCALE?

- Am I really hungry? (Hunger registers between "0" and "4" on the scale.)

- Do I physically need food right now or am I eating for some other reason?

While you are eating, stop and ask yourself:

- Where am I on the HUNGER/FULLNESS SCALE?

- Am I still hungry or do I feel satisfied? (Fullness registers between "6" and "10" on the scale.)

- Could I stop now and save the rest of this food for later?

- Learn to distinguish between satisfied and stuffed.

After you have finished eating, stop and ask yourself:

- Where am I on the fullness side of the scale?

- Have I eaten more than my body needs?

Record your findings by spending a few minutes each day filling in the appropriate column in your FOOD & ACTIVITY JOURNAL. If you practice using the HUNGER/FULLNESS SCALE, checking in with your physical hunger will soon become an automatic part of your eating routine.

Exercise: Set Your Priorities Straight

 "I don't have time for exercise." Sound familiar? Lack of time is the most common reason people give for not exercising. Before you throw in the towel, stop and think for a moment. When you commit to doing something, you MAKE the time for it. If you want to achieve a healthier weight, exercise needs to be a top priority on your list of things to do. Exercise helps you look and feel your best, but it does require making trade-offs. Take a few minutes to reflect on what these would be for you and record them below.

Example:

Benefits of Exercise	Trade-offs
• Looking and feeling better	• Less time for TV
• Less body fat	• Less time for sitting and relaxing
• Reduced stress level	• Initial muscle soreness
• More energy	• Time away from home

Your turn:

Benefits of Exercise	Trade-offs
•	•
•	•
•	•
•	•

Make Room for Fitness

Once you commit to a more active lifestyle, you'll need to *plan* time for your fitness activities each week. Pull out your calendar or daily planner and look at the upcoming week. Note where you have blank spots or free time, even brief periods such as half an hour. Would you be willing to fit a short ten- to fifteen-minute walk into that slot?

Make "appointments" with yourself to exercise. <u>Write them down</u> on your calendar or in your day planner. Honor them just as you would a doctor or dental appointment. If people request this time, tell them: *"I'm sorry I can't do it then. I have an appointment."* They don't need to know that you've made an appointment with yourself!

Making a S.M.A.R.T. Plan

 When it comes to improving our health, we all know what we are supposed to do — eat healthy and move more. It sounds easy enough, but getting started can be tough. A good plan can be a step in the right direction, serving as a personal road map. The key to success — set up a S.M.A.R.T. plan. Effective S.M.A.R.T. plans are. . .

Specific	Be precise about what you expect to achieve.
Measurable	Include amounts, times, days and other milestones for gauging success.
Achievable	Be reasonable; is your plan attainable given what is currently happening in your life?
Relevant	Be sure your plan is meaningful and important to *you.*
Trackable	Record your progress regularly to measure your achievements.

Here is an example of a NOT-SO-S.M.A.R.T. and a S.M.A.R.T. fitness plan:

NOT-SO-S.M.A.R.T. Plan

I haven't been doing any type of activity, so this week I will exercise for an hour every day.

Plan Checklist:

Is it specific?	No, I didn't specify what activity I plan to do or when I intend to do it.
Is it measurable?	Yes, one hour every day.
Is it achievable?	Probably not. Where will I suddenly find a free hour every day for activity? If I've been inactive, a whole hour of activity may be a set-up for a painful experience such as sore muscles or a possible injury.
Is it relevant?	Probably not; sounds like overkill.
Is it trackable?	No, I don't have a plan for keeping a record of my activity.

S.M.A.R.T. Plan

I will walk three days this week (Monday, Wednesday, Friday) for 20 minutes each day. I will do this at 6:00 a.m. before work. This plan will work for me because I enjoy walking and I'm a "morning person." I don't have anyone at home who needs my attention at that time. My neighbor will join me for these walks. We have been walking partners in the past. I will record my minutes of walking in my FOOD & ACTIVITY JOURNAL.

Plan Checklist:

Is it specific?	Yes, walking is the specified activity and it's planned for the a.m.
Is it measurable?	Yes, three days a week for 20 minutes.
Is it achievable?	Yes, I have walked with my neighbor in the past.
Is it relevant?	Yes, walking is an activity I enjoy.
Is it trackable?	Yes, I will record my walking in my FOOD & ACTIVITY JOURNAL.

Throughout this workbook you will be designing S.M.A.R.T. plans for yourself. They will guide you on your path to a healthier lifestyle. Stop and take ten minutes now to set up a S.M.A.R.T. fitness plan for this week (see page 48). The key is to be as specific and realistic as possible.

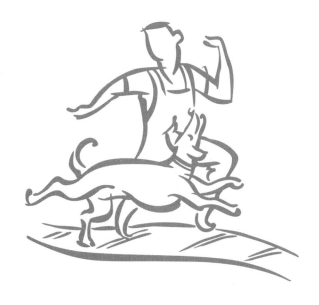

S.M.A.R.T. Fitness Plan for this Week

Specific

What activity(s) will I do?

What time of day would work best?

Measurable

How many days will I exercise?

Which days will I exercise?

How many minutes will I do it for?

Achievable

Is this plan realistic given my schedule this week? (Consider time constraints and available support.)

Relevant

Is this an activity I enjoy?

Can I make it a priority this week?

Trackable

Where will I record my activity?

Skill Practice: Week Two

 Practice may not always make you perfect; however, it does help you focus on your goals and stay committed to changing unhealthy habits. In the upcoming week, focus on the following:

1. **Keep records** — Keep track of your eating habits using one of the following methods.

   ☐ Record food and hunger/fullness cues. (See suggestion.)

   ☐ Record food only.

   ☐ My own tracking system

   (specify): _____

   Suggestion: This week use your FOOD & ACTIVITY JOURNAL to track your body's hunger and fullness levels *each time you eat.* This involves checking in three times during the eating process: once before you begin eating, once in the middle of eating, and once at the end of a meal or snack. Each time ask, "How do I feel? Where am I on the HUNGER/FULLNESS SCALE?" Record only the numbers you get at the *beginning* and *end* of your meal or snack. If this suggestion doesn't work for you, then select another option for tracking your eating habits.

2. **S.M.A.R.T. plan for fitness** — Get moving! Try out the fitness plan you made for yourself this week.

3. **Do a nutrition check** — Select a day from your journal and plug your food choices into the blank Food Pyramid on the next page. See how your food selections match up. Note: If you wish to make additional copies of this pyramid, refer to the Appendix.

> *Reminder:* Don't forget to record your fitness activities in your FOOD & ACTIVITY JOURNAL.

Your Personal Food Pyramid

Instructions: Look at your Food & Activity Journal. Fill in the Food Pyramid according to how many servings of each group you ate. Compare what you ate to the recommended amounts.

Fats, Oils, Sweets

Milk Products
(2–3 servings)

1. _____
2. _____
3. _____

Meat & Alternatives
(2–3 servings)

1. _____
2. _____
3. _____

Vegetables *(3–5 servings)*

1. _____
2. _____
3. _____
4. _____
5. _____

Fruits *(2–4 servings)*

1. _____
2. _____
3. _____
4. _____

Breads, Cereals, Rice, Pasta *(6–11 servings)*

1. _____
2. _____
3. _____
4. _____

5. _____
6. _____
7. _____
8. _____

9. _____
10. _____
11. _____

What changes do you plan to make? _____
_____
_____
_____

FOOD & ACTIVITY JOURNAL

Date:_____

Day: M   Tu   W   Th   F   Sat   Sun

Fitness Activity:

TIME	FEELINGS CHECK	H/F SCALE*	FOOD & DRINK	AMOUNT	CALORIES	FAT (grams)	H/F SCALE*
					Total:	Total:	

*Rate your hunger/fullness on a scale from 0–10: 0 = Empty, 5 = Just Right, 10 = Stuffed

FOOD & ACTIVITY JOURNAL

Date:_____

Day: M   Tu   W   Th   F   Sat   Sun

Fitness Activity:

TIME	FEELINGS CHECK	H/F SCALE*	FOOD & DRINK	AMOUNT	CALORIES	FAT (grams)	H/F SCALE*
					Total:	Total:	

*Rate your hunger/fullness on a scale from 0–10: 0 = Empty, 5 = Just Right, 10 = Stuffed

FOOD & ACTIVITY JOURNAL

Date:_____

Day: M Tu W Th F Sat Sun

Fitness Activity:

TIME	FEELINGS CHECK	H/F SCALE*	FOOD & DRINK	AMOUNT	CALORIES	FAT (grams)	H/F SCALE*
					Total:	Total:	

*Rate your hunger/fullness on a scale from 0–10: 0 = Empty, 5 = Just Right, 10 = Stuffed

FOOD & ACTIVITY JOURNAL

Date:_____

Day: M   Tu   W   Th   F   Sat   Sun

Fitness Activity:

TIME	FEELINGS CHECK	H/F SCALE*	FOOD & DRINK	AMOUNT	CALORIES	FAT (grams)	H/F SCALE*
					Total:	Total:	

*Rate your hunger/fullness on a scale from 0–10: 0 = Empty, 5 = Just Right, 10 = Stuffed

FOOD & ACTIVITY JOURNAL

Date:_____

Day: M   Tu   W   Th   F   Sat   Sun

Fitness Activity:

TIME	FEELINGS CHECK	H/F SCALE*	FOOD & DRINK	AMOUNT	CALORIES	FAT (grams)	H/F SCALE*
					Total:	Total:	

*Rate your hunger/fullness on a scale from 0–10: 0 = Empty, 5 = Just Right, 10 = Stuffed

FOOD & ACTIVITY JOURNAL

Date:_____

Day: M   Tu   W   Th   F   Sat   Sun

Fitness Activity:

TIME	FEELINGS CHECK	H/F SCALE*	FOOD & DRINK	AMOUNT	CALORIES	FAT (grams)	H/F SCALE*
					Total:	Total:	

*Rate your hunger/fullness on a scale from 0–10: 0 = Empty, 5 = Just Right, 10 = Stuffed

FOOD & ACTIVITY JOURNAL

Date:_____

Day: M   Tu   W   Th   F   Sat   Sun

Fitness Activity:	

TIME	FEELINGS CHECK	H/F SCALE*	FOOD & DRINK	AMOUNT	CALORIES	FAT (grams)	H/F SCALE*
					Total:	Total:	

*Rate your hunger/fullness on a scale from 0–10: 0 = Empty, 5 = Just Right, 10 = Stuffed

Up and Running

A habit cannot be tossed out the window — it must be coaxed down the stairs and out the door one step at a time . . .

—*Mark Twain*

You don't have to be perfect in order to make progress. More often than not, progress is two steps forward and one step back. Be patient with yourself while learning new skills.

This Week You Will:

- Reflect over the previous week, noting insights and accomplishments.
- Build support for yourself in living a healthier lifestyle.
- Gain perspective about your expectations.
- Discover where calories come from and how to track them.
- Explore ways to build support for a more active lifestyle.
- Design a personal S.M.A.R.T. plan for food and fitness.

Reflections

Reflect on your FOOD & ACTIVITY JOURNAL

Last week you used the HUNGER/FULLNESS SCALE to track hunger/fullness signals before, during and after eating. What did you learn from this activity?

Reflect on the Food Pyramid

How did your food selections match up? If you need to improve, what are some things you could do?

Reflect on your S.M.A.R.T. fitness plan

How did this plan work for you? Do you plan to use it again, throw it out, or fine-tune it?

Other observations from last week

What worked well for you? What didn't work?

Building Support: Taking Care of Yourself

 We all need a little help at times. When it comes to carrying out our weekly plans, having a little support can often make the difference between thinking and doing. It takes a little work to ask for help, and you may feel uncomfortable at first, but the results are worth it.

The More Safety Lines, the Better!

In a sense, we are like boats bobbing on the water, connected to a dock for safety and stability. This dock is built out of healthy habits. We are linked securely to the dock by one line that represents the support we give ourselves. When the stormy waters of life hit, we can be thrown about and perhaps even severed from the dock if we try to go it alone.

In our desire to make healthful changes or reach new goals, additional lines of support can make the difference. These support lines may come in the form of friends, family or professionals. Thus, when the waters become rough, we will be secured to the dock by not just one line, but many. More lines of support make us more stable and better able to handle life's storms.

Source: Adapted from Byron Kehler, Agape Youth and Family Ministries

---

Support Yourself

Take a moment to identify ways that you would be willing to support yourself. Check off all that apply. Fill in any of your own ideas.

☐ Lighten up on your expectations. Recognize that changing habits is a slow process that takes time. Be patient!

☐ Learn how to say "no, thank you" without feeling guilty.

☐ Don't refer to yourself as "being on a diet." The word "diet" implies deprivation and a temporary way of behaving. Instead, use words like "lifestyle changes" or a "new eating style."

☐ Reward yourself in non-food ways: treat yourself to a new book or magazine, tool or flowers. (See page 78 for a list of non-food rewards.)

☐ Give yourself a mental pat on the back for each positive action or attitude that helps you lead a healthier lifestyle.

☐ Give yourself permission to spend time, energy or money on yourself to:

_____

☐ Other: _____

Support from Others

Now take a minute and think about the support you would like from other people in your life. Read through the list below and check all the boxes that you feel apply to your situation. Feel free to add your own requests to this list.

☐ Please notice and appreciate the healthy changes I am making. Give me praise when you see me taking care of myself by exercising or making healthier food choices.

☐ Support my efforts to exercise: free up my time, give me a piece of equipment, or exercise with me.

☐ Help me stock the house with healthier foods. Make sure that my favorite yogurt, fruits, vegetables, pretzels, popcorn and low-fat crackers are available.

☐ Keep "problem" foods out of the house (foods that I find difficult to resist).

☐ Please refrain from giving me food gifts. Bring me non-food treats instead, like books or flowers.

☐ Stop offering me food. Recognize that if want it, I am capable of getting it for myself.

☐ Recognize that I am in charge of my own life. Never mention diets or my weight. Stop being the food police — don't tell me what to eat and what not to eat.

☐ Please do not eat junk food in front of me; eat these foods when I am not around.

☐ Stop nagging or blaming me for being overweight and stop comparing me to thin people.

☐ _____

☐ _____

Asking for Support

Asking for Help: Part One

If you don't feel comfortable asking other people for help or if you're out of practice, don't panic! Use this simple, five-step plan as a guide to securing the support that you need.

Step 1: Respectfully acknowledge the person you are asking for help.

Ideas:
- Thank the person for listening.
- Acknowledge the person's busy schedule.
- Express gratefulness for help in past situations.

Step 2: Tell the person what you need.

Step 3: Tell the person how you would like to be supported. Be specific.

Step 4: Stay flexible and be willing to negotiate.

This is especially important if your request involves time or money. Find a solution that works for both of you.

Step 5: Thank the person for their support.

> *Note:* If you can't think of someone to ask for support, continue this exercise and use the worksheet to ask yourself for more support.

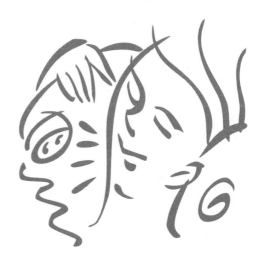

Asking for Help: Part Two

When it comes to asking others for support, practice what you want to say first. You'll feel more at ease and you're more likely to be heard. Writing your thoughts down on paper is an ideal way to do this. Read through the following example to see how easy and effective this approach can be.

BUILDING SUPPORT WORKSHEET

(Example of Asking Another Person for Support.)

A person I would like support from:

My husband

In what way(s) do I want this person to help me?

I would like more time for exercise.

Making the Request for Help: BE SPECIFIC!
(Practice in writing how you will say it in person.)

Step 1: Respectfully acknowledge the person you are asking for help.

I know this is a busy time for you at work and I appreciate all the time you have been spending with the kids.

Step 2: Tell the person what you need.

I am trying to make more time in my schedule for exercise and I would appreciate your help.

Step 3: Tell the person how you would like to be supported. Be specific.

Would you be willing to get the kids up and off to school on Mondays, Wednesdays and Fridays so that I could get in a morning walk before I go to work?

Step 4: Stay flexible; be willing to negotiate. This is important if your request involves time or money. Find a solution that works for both of you.

If you do this for me during the week, I will get up with the kids and get them going on the weekend days.

Step 5: Thank the person for their support.

I appreciate your willingness to help me out. Thank you!

BUILDING SUPPORT WORKSHEET

(Example of Asking Yourself for More Support.)

A person I would like support from:

Myself.

In what way(s) do I want this person to help me?

To self: Stop making judgments about my food choices.

Making the Request for Help: BE SPECIFIC!
(Practice in writing how you will say it.)

Step 1: Respectfully acknowledge the person you are asking for help in this case, yourself.

I know I'm trying to be more aware of what I eat, but labeling food as "good" or "bad" just makes me feel deprived and rebellious.

Step 2: Tell the person what you need.

I need to talk to myself in a more gentle and encouraging manner.

I need to focus on all the healthy foods I like to eat instead of focusing on all the foods "I shouldn't eat."

Step 3: Tell the person how you would like to be supported. Be specific.

I'll quit labeling foods as "good" and "bad." I won't withhold or deprive myself of my favorite foods (chocolate and cookies). I'll purchase these foods in small amounts and enjoy them.

I'll encourage myself with a mental pat on the back when I make healthy food choices.

Step 4: Stay flexible; be willing to negotiate. This is important if your request involves time or money. Find a solution that works for both of you.

I'll give myself permission to spend a little extra money on healthy foods I like (fresh pineapple, shrimp, baked potato chips).

Step 5: Thank the person for their support.

I'll acknowledge myself every time I'm positive and encouraging rather than critical and judgmental.

Asking for Help: Part Three

Now it's your turn to practice asking someone else (or yourself) for support. The first step is to fill out the BUILDING SUPPORT WORKSHEET below. This activity will take about five to 10 minutes. Practice in writing asking for what you need and explaining how this person can help you the most. Be as clear and precise as you can.

BUILDING SUPPORT WORKSHEET

A person I would like support from:

In what way(s) do I want this person to help me?

Making the Request for Help: BE SPECIFIC!

Step 1: Respectfully acknowledge the person you are asking for help.

Step 2: Tell the person what you need.

Step 3: Tell the person how you would like to be supported. Be specific.

Step 4: Stay flexible; be willing to negotiate. This is important if your request involves time or money. Find a solution that works for both of you.

Step 5: Thank the person for their support.

Once you've finished writing down what you want to say, ask a supportive family member or friend to role-play with you. Just speaking the words out loud a few times can help you when the time really comes. If you don't have a family member or friend to assist you, try speaking it out loud while standing in front of a mirror. You may feel uncomfortable or even silly, but if you get the support you need in the end, it's well worth it!

When Others Aren't Supportive

You won't always receive the support you desire. It's a tough fact of life. When others aren't supportive, you still need to be able to cope. Here are some suggestions:

- Speak up for your needs when you feel sabotaged.

- Avoid or distance yourself from certain people or situations, or anticipate them and develop a plan in advance.

- Contact other people who can help when you don't know how to deal with a situation. Helpful support may come from friends, family members, counselors, neighbors, colleagues, health professionals, and clergy.

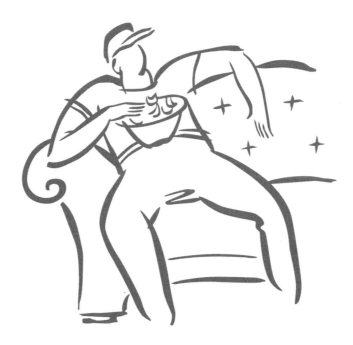

Facts of Life: Taming Your Expectations

Working toward a healthier lifestyle is like taking a journey down a long and winding road. You know you will encounter hills and valleys, as well as a few other surprises, along the way. Do you remember the children's game of Chutes & Ladders? Wouldn't it be nice if you always had a ladder handy to help yourself over the tough spots? When you hit a difficult patch on the road to good health, lean on these "ladders" to keep yourself moving forward.

- **Changing habits is slow going** — It takes time and patience. In fact, it can take up to a YEAR before a new behavior or habit becomes automatic.

- **Progress, not perfection** — Acknowledge your successes, however small they may be. There is no one "right" way to do things.

- **The 80/20 rule** — The idea is not to be perfect, but to make healthier choices more often. Strive to make wise choices 80% of the time; go easy on yourself the other 20% of the time. If you do, you will head in the right direction without feeling guilty or deprived.

- **Be gentle with yourself while establishing new habits** — Suspend your inner critical voice. Strive to find something positive in every situation. Encourage yourself and move forward. For example, instead of berating yourself if you overeat at dinner, just skip dessert. You can always have it tomorrow.

- **Recognize that setbacks are part of progress** — If you stumble (and you will), remember your past successes and immediately plan for the future.

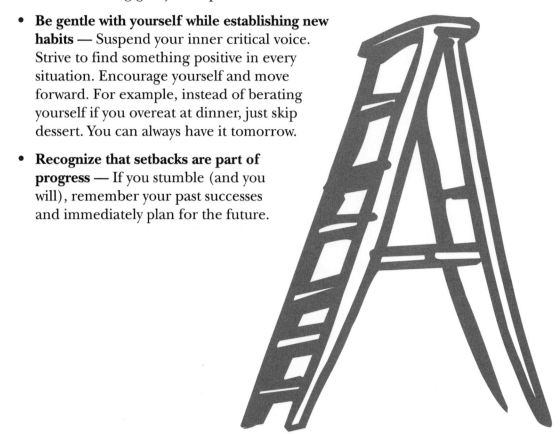

Achieving a Healthy Weight

Your weight is unique, just like your fingerprints. Your genes and your lifestyle choices influence it. Don't strive to achieve an ideal body weight, size or shape — it doesn't exist! Aim to reach a healthy weight instead. A weight you look and feel your best at, and one you don't have to starve or deprive yourself to maintain.

Good health, after all, entails more than just reaching a certain number on the scale. It's a state of physical, mental and social well-being. You can't change your genes, but you can change the way you move and the foods you choose to eat. *Smart CHOICES* will help you concentrate on changing unhealthy habits into healthier choices.

How often should I weigh myself?

How often you choose to step on a scale is up to you, but take your personal reactions into account. If you hop on the scale and the number is up, how does this affect you? Is your day ruined? Do you berate yourself? If you answered "yes" to either of these questions, the number on the scale is too emotionally loaded for you. Hopping on and off the scale every day may be more of a hindrance than help.

On the other hand, if you haven't weighed yourself in years, you may be in denial about your weight. When you don't weigh yourself, you may disconnect from your body. This sense of detachment can affect your ability to take responsibility for your body and give it the care that it needs and deserves.

Weighing yourself too often or not at all can hinder your goal of achieving a healthy weight. Try weighing yourself once a week. Be objective when it comes to the scale. Your weight provides only one form of feedback and it doesn't always accurately reflect your body's changes. For example, it's possible to gain muscle weight from regular workouts while losing body fat without seeing any change on the scale. Day-to-day fluctuations in body fluids also influence this number. The scale doesn't say, "You are up two pounds today because you're retaining fluid," or "You are down one pound today because you're dehydrated." It's wise to keep these numbers in perspective.

Body Shape: Apple or Pear?

Does your weight increase your risk for health problems? Part of the answer lies in the shape of your body and where you tend to store fat. A tendency to store excess fat in the upper body or belly — an apple shape — puts you at higher risk for heart disease, high blood pressure and diabetes. Excess weight stored in the hips and thighs — a pear shape — appears to be less risky healthwise.

Calories Count

 Calories, calories, calories. Everybody talks about them, but you never actually see one. Where do they come from and why should you keep an eye on how many you consume? Calories are a measure of the energy available from food. This energy fuels your body the same way gas fuels a car. Calories from low-nutrient foods are like inexpensive gas. They leave you feeling sluggish, weak and low on energy. Calories from "high-octane" or nutrient-rich foods enable you to feel strong and full of energy and to function at your best. Rely on the Food Guide Pyramid and food labels to help you select "high-octane" foods.

Where do calories come from?

You don't have to look very far to find where calories come from. All the foods you eat, as well as most beverages, provide calories. Three major nutrients found in food — protein, carbohydrate and fat — as well as alcohol supply calories or energy that your body uses. Take a close look at the numbers to see how they stack up against each other.

1 gram of carbohydrate = 4 calories

1 gram of protein = 4 calories

1 gram of fat = 9 calories

1 gram of alcohol = 7 calories

Did you notice that fat and alcohol weigh in on the heavy end? They supply approximately twice as many calories per gram as proteins and carbohydrates.

Nearly all foods contain a mixture of carbohydrate, protein and fat. For example, we often view meat and cheese as protein foods. Yet a one-ounce slice of cheese provides 9 grams of fat and only 7 grams of protein. Cheese is actually more fat (74% of its total calories) than protein (25% of its total calories). Take a look at steak; an 8-ounce portion of prime rib provides 67 grams of fat and 53 grams of protein—a whopping 73% of total calories from fat. To learn more about the carbohydrate, protein and fat in a particular food, check the Nutrition Facts section on food labels.

No matter what kind of food you eat — even healthy foods like complex carbohydrates — if you eat more than your body needs for fuel, your body converts the extra calories into fat.

How many calories do you need?

Your calorie needs depend on a lot of different factors, such as your age, gender (men generally need more than women do), activity level, dieting history (chronic dieters seem to need fewer calories), body composition (how much muscle you have versus fat), and your genetic makeup. Everyone is different! No hard and fast rules exist for determining the exact number of calories that you need. In fact, your calorie or energy requirements can vary greatly from day to day. For example, a mountain climber burns more calories hiking in cold, snowy weather than in hot, dry weather.

Calculating Calories to Lose Weight

Use these two simple methods to *estimate* your caloric needs.

Method #1:
Track the number of calories you eat for three days; total the calories each day, and then add the three days together and divide by three to obtain your average caloric intake. Watch your weight over this same time period. If it remains the same, you have a good estimate of the number of calories you need to maintain your weight. To lose weight, subtract 20% (but NOT more) from your "maintenance" calorie level. For example, if you maintain your weight on 2400 calories, you would need to eat approximately 1900 calories to lose weight.

Method #2:
Use the rule of 12. To lose weight, multiply your realistic target weight (not your current weight) by 12. For example, if you want to weigh 150 pounds, you would need to eat 1800 calories per day (150 x 12 = 1800). To maintain your weight, multiply your current weight by 13 to 15. (This range reflects differences in physical activity levels.)

Tracking Your Calories

Think about calories as you do money. You have a limited amount, so spend it wisely. When you track your calories, it helps you see how you spend them. For example, what types of food provide most of your calories? How do your food choices compare with the Food Guide Pyramid recommendations? Do you tend to graze throughout the day or inhale most of your calories at night? Do you eat more or fewer calories when you eat at home compared to a night on the town? How about during the week compared to weekends? Keeping track of your calories can help you answer all of these questions, plus more.

Accurate Tracking

Before you begin recording your calories, consider these helpful tips.

Size Up Your Servings — You won't get very far tracking calories if you don't have a good handle on serving sizes. There can be a big difference between a "serving" as listed on a food label and the amount that actually ends up on your plate. For example, a package of rice lists 1/2 cup (for 100 calories) as the reference serving, but you may easily eat one cup — 200 calories or twice the food label "serving."

Check In With Reality — You don't have to weigh and measure every morsel. Check portions of your favorite foods instead. For example, if you generally start your day by eating a bowl of cereal, pour the cereal into the bowl as you normally would. Remove the cereal from the bowl and measure it with a measuring cup. How much do you really eat? Try this with another food. Measure out a teaspoon of margarine. What does it look like and how does it compare to what you normally use? Use measuring spoons to check on mayonnaise, salad dressing and peanut butter; dry measuring cups for cooked pasta and rice; a liquid measuring cup for beverages. If you don't have a kitchen scale, you may find it a challenge to measure meat and cheese. Use the following guidelines to guess-timate your portions.

    1 ounce = book of matches
    3 ounces = deck of cards

Don't Wait — The longer you wait to write in your FOOD & ACTIVITY JOURNAL, the more likely you are to forget what you ate. As soon as you finish eating, write down at least the foods you consumed (including serving sizes). You can look up and record the calories at a later time. To make the job easier, save the food labels off packaged foods. Sometimes you may know what you will be eating ahead of time. Write these foods down beforehand, check back and make corrections after you've eaten.

If you feel overwhelmed

Once again, if you find yourself making a judgment about every morsel that passes between your lips, STOP! You are not on a diet. A FOOD & ACTIVITY JOURNAL simply helps you become more aware of your eating and exercise habits. Make this JOURNAL a tool for learning. If you choose not to track calories, you will still gain a lot by simply writing down the foods you eat and estimating your portion sizes. Knowledge is power. The more you know about your current eating habits, the better prepared you will be to make changes in the future.

Warning! Never slip below 1200 to 1400 calories a day. Eating too few calories actually slows down your body's metabolism as it attempts to ward off starvation. Besides, if you go too low, you won't have enough energy to remain physically active.

Support for a More Active Lifestyle

 To be more active on a regular basis, build a support system so you don't have to go it alone. For example, think of a person who may be willing to exercise with you. Having an exercise partner makes all the difference for some people — especially at 6 a.m. or after a tough day at the office.

If you enjoy exercising with others, how will you obtain that support?

Ideas: Enlist an exercise partner (neighbor, family member, friends at work), take a class, join a swimming or fitness center.

Next, ask yourself what other people could do to make it easier for you to have more time in your schedule to exercise. Here are several possible scenarios that might give you some ideas:

- Maybe your boss would be willing to let you start work earlier in the day so that you could leave a little early to catch a fitness class across town.

- Family members could help out with dinner preparations so you could squeeze in a 20-minute walk before dinner.

- Perhaps your spouse would trade time with you in the care of your young children — you get designated time for your fitness activity, and your spouse receives designated time for herself/himself.

In what way(s) could you rearrange your schedule to better support your fitness plans? Whom and what would this involve?

Making a S.M.A.R.T. Food Plan

 Last week you made a S.M.A.R.T. fitness plan. This week you'll add a S.M.A.R.T. food plan to the picture. Think of one eating habit you can change for the better and make a S.M.A.R.T. food plan on the following page. For ideas, see examples listed below or refer to your Reflections on page 32 (items listed under "ready and willing to change now").

S.M.A.R.T. FOOD PLAN EXAMPLES

Eat vegetables two times a day for five days this week.

Try one new low-fat recipe this week.

Take fruit to work for my afternoon snack at least three days this week.

Limit the number of times I eat red meat for lunch and dinner to ____ times this week.

Order salad dressing on the side when I go out to restaurants this week.

Cut down on fat by eating toast and rolls with honey or jam in place of butter this week.

Eat breakfast five days this week.

Say "no, thank you" at least once this week to food offered to me.

Preplan my dinner meal at least four days this week.

Practice leaving food on my plate by leaving at least one bite of food on my dinner plate at least four days this week.

Practice slowing down my pace of eating by making dinner meals last at least 20 minutes for at least four days this week.

Choose not to eat any fried foods this week.

Limit the amount of wine I drink this week to ____ four-ounce glasses.

S.M.A.R.T. FOOD PLAN

Specific
What will I work on?

Eating a healthy snack in the afternoon at work.

Measurable
How many days will I do it for?

4 days

Which days will I target? (weekdays, weekends)

Monday through Thursday

Achievable
Is this plan realistic? Reasonable?

Yes, if I buy healthy snacks at the grocery store on the weekend.

Relevant
Will changing this eating habit make a difference in my health?

Yes. If I don't plan ahead for a healthy snack at work then I get too hungry and I overeat when I get home.

Trackable
How will I monitor this behavior?

Food & Activity Journal

My S.M.A.R.T. Plans for this Week

Stop and take a few minutes to set up a S.M.A.R.T. fitness plan for yourself this week. It may be the same or different from last week's plan. Add a S.M.A.R.T. food plan. Remember to be as specific and realistic as possible.

S.M.A.R.T. FITNESS PLAN	S.M.A.R.T. FOOD PLAN
Specific What activity(s) will I do? Time of day? (a.m. or p.m.)	Specific What will I work on?
Measurable How many days will I exercise? Which days will I exercise? How many minutes will I do it for?	Measurable How many days will I do it for? Which days will I target? (weekdays, weekends)
Achievable Is this plan realistic? Reasonable?	Achievable Is this plan realistic? Reasonable?
Relevant Is this an activity I enjoy? Can I make it a priority this week?	Relevant Will changing this eating habit make a difference in my health?
Trackable Where will I record my activity?	Trackable How will I monitor this behavior?

Skill Practice: Week Three

Take advantage of these opportunities to practice and enhance your skills this week.

1. **Keep records** — Keep track of your eating habits using one of the following methods.

   ☐ Record food and calories. (See suggestion.)

   ☐ Record food only.

   ☐ Record food and hunger/fullness cues.

   ☐ Use the Food Pyramid for a nutrition check. (See Appendix.)

   ☐ My own tracking system

   (specify): _____

   Suggestion: In the week ahead, record everything that you eat and drink in your **FOOD & ACTIVITY JOURNAL**. Track your calories in the space provided. Use information available on food labels and the **CALORIE & FAT COUNTER** (see pages 255-280) to determine calorie counts. If this suggestion doesn't work for you, then select another option for tracking your eating habits.

2. **S.M.A.R.T. plans** — Follow the fitness and food plans you made for yourself this week.

3. **Asking for support** — This week, ask at least one person (or yourself) to support your efforts at becoming a healthier person.

Reminder: Don't forget to record your fitness activities in your **FOOD & ACTIVITY JOURNAL**.

Non-Food Rewards

Having a night out alone or with a friend/spouse
Going to a movie
Spending an afternoon at the beach or in the mountains
Getting a manicure or massage
Buying a new book or magazine
Taking a nap
Sleeping in on a weekend morning
Taking a hot bath (with candlelight and/or bath fragrances)
Recreational activity (golf, bowling, skiing, etc.)
Going out dancing
Visiting with a friend
Buying fresh-cut flowers
Taking a walk or hike
Playing a musical instrument
Taking the car to be cleaned
Listening to favorite music
Spending time on a craft, hobby or fun project
Shopping or browsing in a favorite store or area of town
Setting the table with linen, china, etc.
Playing with children
Building a fire in the fireplace
Purchasing a favorite perfume or aftershave
Calling someone special long-distance
Attending a play, concert or athletic event
Buying new makeup or a pair of fun new socks
Sitting in the sunshine
New hairstyle
Playing a game (crossword puzzles, cards, etc.)
Writing (letters, journal, etc.)
Playing with pets
Soaking in a hot tub
Extra time for reading

Your ideas:

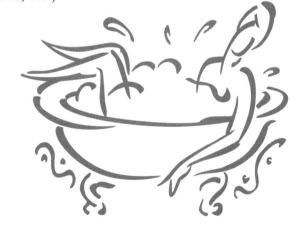

FOOD & ACTIVITY JOURNAL

Date:_____

Day: M   Tu   W   Th   F   Sat   Sun

Fitness Activity:	

TIME	FEELINGS CHECK	H/F SCALE*	FOOD & DRINK	AMOUNT	CALORIES	FAT (grams)	H/F SCALE*
					Total:	Total:	

*Rate your hunger/fullness on a scale from 0–10: 0 = Empty, 5 = Just Right, 10 = Stuffed

FOOD & ACTIVITY JOURNAL

Date:_____

Day: M   Tu   W   Th   F   Sat   Sun

Fitness Activity:

TIME	FEELINGS CHECK	H/F SCALE*	FOOD & DRINK	AMOUNT	CALORIES	FAT (grams)	H/F SCALE*
					Total:	Total:	

*Rate your hunger/fullness on a scale from 0–10: 0 = Empty, 5 = Just Right, 10 = Stuffed

FOOD & ACTIVITY JOURNAL

Date:_____

Day: M   Tu   W   Th   F   Sat   Sun

Fitness Activity:

TIME	FEELINGS CHECK	H/F SCALE*	FOOD & DRINK	AMOUNT	CALORIES	FAT (grams)	H/F SCALE*
					Total:	Total:	

*Rate your hunger/fullness on a scale from 0–10: 0 = Empty, 5 = Just Right, 10 = Stuffed

FOOD & ACTIVITY JOURNAL

Date:_____

Day: M   Tu   W   Th   F   Sat   Sun

Fitness Activity:

TIME	FEELINGS CHECK	H/F SCALE*	FOOD & DRINK	AMOUNT	CALORIES	FAT (grams)	H/F SCALE*
					Total:	Total:	

*Rate your hunger/fullness on a scale from 0–10: 0 = Empty, 5 = Just Right, 10 = Stuffed

FOOD & ACTIVITY JOURNAL

Date:_____

Day: M   Tu   W   Th   F   Sat   Sun

Fitness Activity:	

TIME	FEELINGS CHECK	H/F SCALE*	FOOD & DRINK	AMOUNT	CALORIES	FAT (grams)	H/F SCALE*
					Total:	Total:	

*Rate your hunger/fullness on a scale from 0–10: 0 = Empty, 5 = Just Right, 10 = Stuffed

FOOD & ACTIVITY JOURNAL

Date:_____

Day: M Tu W Th F Sat Sun

Fitness Activity:

TIME	FEELINGS CHECK	H/F SCALE*	FOOD & DRINK	AMOUNT	CALORIES	FAT (grams)	H/F SCALE*
					Total:	Total:	

*Rate your hunger/fullness on a scale from 0–10: 0 = Empty, 5 = Just Right, 10 = Stuffed

FOOD & ACTIVITY JOURNAL

Date:_____

Day: M   Tu   W   Th   F   Sat   Sun

Fitness Activity:

TIME	FEELINGS CHECK	H/F SCALE*	FOOD & DRINK	AMOUNT	CALORIES	FAT (grams)	H/F SCALE*
					Total:	Total:	

*Rate your hunger/fullness on a scale from 0–10: 0 = Empty, 5 = Just Right, 10 = Stuffed

Fit and Healthy

The healthy choices you make on a daily basis can really pay off when it comes to managing your weight. Think about all the positive choices you can make, such as packing a lunch instead of going out for fast food, or taking leftovers home from a restaurant. They may seem insignificant, but big improvements can come from small changes. Your job is to acknowledge the positive choices that you make and give yourself a pat on the back. Small changes, after all, form the foundation of a healthier lifestyle.

> This Week You Will:
>
> - Reflect over the previous week, noting insights and accomplishments.
> - Learn about the elements of a good fitness plan and F.I.T. guidelines for exercise.
> - Learn about fat in your diet, such as how to spot hidden fat in foods and some easy ways to track and budget fat in your diet.
> - Take a food label tour and unlock the secrets of nutrition labeling.
> - Design a personal S.M.A.R.T. plan for food and fitness.

Reflections

Reflect on building support

What opportunities did you have to ask for support? Whom did you ask? How did it go for you?

Reflect on your FOOD & ACTIVITY JOURNAL

Last week's suggestion was to track calories in your FOOD & ACTIVITY JOURNAL. If you did this activity, what did you learn? How did you spend your calories? Consider taste and nutrition.

Reflect on your S.M.A.R.T. plans

How did these plans work for you? Do you plan to use them again, throw them out or fine-tune them?

Other observations from last week

What worked well for you? What didn't work?

The Fitness Formula

 By now, you've hopefully found some activities you enjoy doing and you're up and moving. You may even be enjoying some of the more immediate rewards of being active — better sleep, less stress and more energy. If you make the commitment to remain active, you'll reap even more benefits over time, like building muscle and losing body fat.

The Elements of a Good Fitness Program

Being fit doesn't require that you take an aerobics class or sweat in the gym seven days a week. But if your goal is to get in shape and lose body fat, you need to come up with some sort of fitness program. Make it your own. Find activities that you enjoy and that fit into your schedule. Whatever you choose, be consistent. You won't reap the long-term rewards of exercise if you don't keep it up.

Keep the following key components in mind as you develop your own fitness program:

- **Endurance or aerobic activity** — *burns fat, increases stamina*

  Aerobic exercise is a nonstop activity that increases your heart rate and uses large muscle groups. The following activities qualify on both counts: fast walking, swimming, bicycling, group fitness classes and roller blading.

- **Flexibility** — *prevents injury, keeps body limber*

  Flexibility refers to stretching exercises that enable your joints to move freely through a full range of motion. Stretching is done after your body is warmed up, usually at the end of a workout. It is a slow, comfortable movement that is held for at least 10-30 seconds. Never bounce, and remember to breathe.

- **Muscular strength** — *improves strength, prevents injury, supports good posture*

  Strengthening exercises consist of activities that use resistance to improve muscle tone and power. Examples of strengthening activities are weight lifting and calisthenics (abdominal crunches, push-ups, pull-ups, etc.). The American College of Sports Medicine recommends strength training at least twice a week, in workouts that can take as little as 15 minutes per session.

Aerobic F.I.T.ness

All physical activity burns calories. But if you want to burn fat and calories and strengthen your heart in the most efficient way, choose aerobic activities. You may be wondering about how much, how often and how hard you have to exercise to get these benefits. You'll find the answers in the following F.I.T. (frequency, intensity, time) guidelines:

Frequency — how often?

Here's some great news — any exercise is better than none at all. If you're just starting out, begin with the number of days that works for you. Gradually increase as you build your fitness level. Work up to being active four to six times a week. The more active you are, the more calories you'll burn. It's better for your body if you exercise a little each day instead of a lot once or twice a week. For example, a 15-minute walk five days a week is better than one 75-minute walk once a week.

Intensity — how hard?

Low- to moderate-level exercise at a steady pace burns more fat than a higher level of activity that leaves you so breathless you can only keep it up for a few minutes. Your body needs oxygen in order to burn fat. When you exercise at an out-of-breath level you burn less fat. Exercise at the right level by using the following chart to help you monitor your body's signals during exercise.

PHYSICAL INDICATORS	SHOULD BE	SHOULD NOT BE
Breathing	Breathing deeply, able to talk but not sing	Gasping for breath; unable to talk
Body Temperature	Feeling warm all over	Overheated
Perspiration	Perspiring lightly	Feeling cold and clammy
Fatigue Level	Invigorated	Exhausted

Time — how long?

Always begin by warming up for five minutes. This means you should start out slowly and gradually increase your pace until your heart is beating faster. Continue until you perspire lightly, yet are still able to talk. When you've reached this level, you've hit your aerobic target zone. Keep your heart rate at this level for a minimum of 20 minutes. Obviously, beginners need to work up to this level gradually. At the end of your aerobic workout, slow your pace over a five- to 10-minute period, letting your heart rate gradually return to normal. Be kind to your muscles and stretch afterwards. Stretching helps prevent muscle stiffness and soreness the next day.

If You Need Help

If you find yourself stuck or unsure about what to do about your fitness routine, you may want to seek additional support. Here are some ideas to help you move forward:

- Hire a qualified personal fitness trainer for a couple of hours. This person will assess your fitness level and set you up with an individualized fitness plan. You can find fitness trainers in clubs, recreational centers, the YMCA or the phone book.

- Register for a fitness class: low-impact aerobics, chair fitness or water aerobics.

- Join a local recreation center, the YMCA or a club. Look for a facility that is convenient, comfortable, and has a professionally trained staff.

- Purchase an exercise video produced by a fitness specialist, not a TV star. Before you spend any money, try renting or borrowing a few from your local video store or library first.

Use it or lose it — it's never too late!

As you grow older, you will lose muscle if you don't use it. Since muscle is metabolically active (burns calories), a decrease in muscle mass results in a decline in metabolism. The good news — you can experience the benefits of exercise at any age. Research studies show that even people ages 90+ respond to strength training programs. So it's never too late to start moving!

Fat — How Low Do You Need to Go?

 Make an effort to trim the fat in your diet. Your heart and your waistline will thank you. Here's the "skinny" on fat:

- Gram for gram, fat delivers twice as many calories as protein or carbohydrates do. Reducing the amount of fat you eat can lead to a big savings in calories.

- A diet high in fat is linked to heart disease and certain types of cancer.

- Fat is fattening. Calories from fat are more easily converted into body fat than the calories from protein or carbohydrates.

Measuring Fat

Fat Grams

Take a look at any food label. The amount of fat present in a food appears in grams (g). To compare the fat content of one product to another, refer to the grams of fat per serving. *Reference:* 1 teaspoon of fat or oil = 5 grams of fat.

Percent of Calories from Fat

You can also determine how much fat is in a particular day's or week's worth of food by calculating the percentage of calories that come from fat. (You will learn how to do this shortly.)

How low should you go?

Most health experts agree that Americans should eat less fat. But opinions vary on how low-fat we should go. Take a look at the range of recommendations.

% Calories from Fat

10-15%	20-25%	30%	33-38%	40%+
• Pritikin • Ornish	*Smart CHOICES*	• American Heart Assoc. • National Cancer Institute	Average American Diet	Not Recommended

Less than 10% Calories from Fat:

Here's a case when less is not better. Fat is an essential nutrient, and you can harm your health by eating too little of it.

10-15% Calories from Fat:

The Pritikin and Ornish diets were developed by two physicians to prevent heart disease and possibly even reverse advanced heart disease in some people. Extremely low in fat and nearly vegetarian, these diets require you to constantly monitor the foods you eat. Some health professionals view these diets as rigid and unrealistic for the average person.

20-25% Calories from Fat:

This is a reasonable approach if you want to reach and maintain a healthy weight. This approach also reduces your risk of health problems and you don't have to give up all your favorite foods. Remember, the goal is to lower the fat in your diet without sacrificing good taste or nutrition.

30% Calories from Fat:

Both the National Cancer Institute and the American Heart Association (AHA) recommend that healthy people reduce their fat intake to less than 30% of total calories, which is a step in the right direction. If you already have heart disease, the AHA recommends reducing your fat intake even further to 25% of total calories.

Use this handy chart to guide you in balancing your fat budget.

CALORIES PER DAY	RECOMMENDED TOTAL FAT GRAMS PER DAY*	TYPICAL AMERICAN DIET: TOTAL FAT GRAMS PER DAY**
1200	30 or fewer	50
1400	35 or fewer	60
1600	40 or fewer	70
1800	50 or fewer	75
2000	55 or fewer	85
2200	60 or fewer	90
2400	65 or fewer	100

*Based on 20-25% Calories from Fat. Numbers are approximate.

**Based on 38% Calories from Fat. Numbers are approximate.

Example: If you eat approximately 1800 calories a day, you would strive to eat 50 grams of fat or less a day.

There's nothing magical about these numbers. Use them as guidelines as you work toward your goal of healthy, low-fat eating. When you evaluate your options regarding the fat in your diet, think in terms of the climate vs. the weather. The climate is your overall fat intake, over a month, for instance. The weather is the day-to-day variation. Some days will be unseasonably rainy or unseasonably dry. The same rings true about the amount of fat you eat — some days you'll be a little over your fat budget and some days a little under.

Where's the Fat?

Some fats are so obvious, they don't even try to hide, such as butter on toast. Others, however, are sneaky and more difficult to detect. Look at the ingredient listing and Nutrition Facts sections on food labels to discover hidden fats.

Visible Fats: Margarine, butter, oil, lard, salad dressing, mayonnaise, sour cream, cream, cream cheese, gravy and cream sauce.

Hidden Fats: Meats, cheese, whole milk, eggs, ice cream, nuts, seeds, coconut, chips, candy bars, pastries, croissants, scones, muffins, doughnuts and other baked goods, olives, avocado, fast food and fried food.

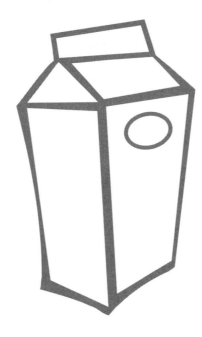

Trimming the Fat

The goal is to cut down on fat, not eliminate it. A low-fat diet is not a fat-free diet. A little fat can make a big difference in taste and nutrition. For example, you would be better off eating a salad with a small amount of regular or reduced-fat salad dressing than to forgo it because you despise fat-free salad dressing.

Ten Tips for Trimming Fat

1. Read food labels and compare different brands by looking at the grams of fat per serving from the Nutrition Facts section of the label.

2. Full-fat cheeses contain more fat than many cuts of red meat! Select reduced-fat cheese (6 grams of fat or less per ounce) or low-fat cheese (3 grams of fat or less per ounce) instead. Skimp on fat, but not taste, by mixing a higher-fat cheese with low-fat or fat-free cheese in your favorite recipes.

3. Cut down on the amount of fat you put on foods: margarine, butter, cream cheese, sour cream, mayonnaise and salad dressing. Switch to lower-fat products when you bake and cook — you won't miss the taste.

4. Limit meat and poultry servings to the size of a deck of cards. Eat more dishes that feature meat as a condiment, not the star player, such as soups, casseroles, stir-fries and shish kebabs.

5. Choose lower-fat dairy products. If you haven't already made the switch, work your way down to skim or 1% milk. Try different brands; each has its own flavor.

6. At mealtime, fill two-thirds of your plate with grains, fruits and vegetables and the other one-third with meat, fish or poultry.

7. Build meals around skinless poultry, fish, shellfish, beans, grains and pasta. These foods contain much less fat than most cuts of meat. As a rule of thumb for meat, cuts with the words "round" or "loin" in the name are generally the leanest, such as round steak, sirloin and tenderloin.

8. Get in the "scraping" habit. When using higher-fat spreads such as margarine, peanut butter, mayonnaise and cream cheese, scrape, don't frost, your bread or bagel. Even some of the "light" versions of these products still carry a significant amount of fat.

9. Try applebutter, honey or jam as a tasty alternative to margarine and butter on your bread or toast.

10. Remember the golden rule you learned in kindergarten — always share. This advice definitely applies to luscious desserts. Just think, a piece of white chocolate cheesecake provides only half the fat and calories when you share it with a friend!

Tracking Your Fat

If you're curious about the amount of fat that you eat, try tracking it in your FOOD & ACTIVITY JOURNAL. You may be surprised at what you find!

- Write down everything you eat or drink. Do this immediately after (or even before) each meal or snack so you don't forget.

- Estimate your serving size. It may be worthwhile to do a reality check and weigh and measure a few items.

- Record the grams of fat for each food/drink item. If you can't find the grams of fat on the food label, refer to the CALORIE & FAT COUNTER.

- At the end of the day, total your fat grams. How does your total compare with the recommended range?

- If you want to know your overall percent of calories from fat for a day, you'll also need to track your calories. To calculate this percentage, use the formula listed below.

Calculating % Calories from Fat:

Step 1: Total grams of fat x 9 calories = calories from fat

Step 2: Calories from fat ÷ total calories x 100 = % calories from fat

Facts of Life: Real Food for Real People

 We live in a world of fat-free everything: cookies, cakes, potato chips, mayonnaise, salad dressings, dairy products, etc. You name it and it most likely comes with little or no fat. Take a few minutes and think about the difference between real food and some of the fake foods now available in supermarkets. Who really enjoys fat-free rubbery cheese?

Food is our body's fuel. We run best on high-octane fuel, such as crusty whole-grain bread, barbecued chicken, spicy black bean burritos, crispy apples, and creamy yogurt topped with fresh berries. These foods nourish our bodies and give us the energy to do the things we like to do. We eat not only to fulfill our physical needs, but also to satisfy cultural and emotional needs as well. Could you imagine Thanksgiving without the turkey or a birthday party without a cake?

Fat-free foods can definitely play a part in your overall effort to lose weight, but consuming them won't make up for a lack of physical activity or extra calories from too-generous servings.

Keeping that in mind, which of the following low-fat lunches do you find more nourishing?

Meal #1   Box of fat-free cookies and a diet pop

Meal #2   Turkey sandwich on whole grain bread, crispy apple and a low-fat coffee latté

Fat-free desserts and chips may have a place in your diet, but strive to eat them with real food, not in place of it. Also, don't be fooled into thinking that all fat-free foods are healthier or that they contain fewer calories because they have less fat. Fat-free cookies, for example, often contain the same number of calories as regular cookies; the fat has simply been replaced with more sugar.

Fake Fat: A Good Choice?

Olean, the trade name for olestra, is a calorie-free fat substitute currently used in some brands of snack foods like potato chips, corn chips, tortilla chips and crackers.

What is olestra?

Olestra is a synthesized compound (not naturally occurring) made by combining everyday ingredients — vegetable oil and table sugar. Olestra's molecules are too large to be digested as it passes through the stomach and intestines. Since it can't be absorbed, it adds no fat or calories to the foods that are made with it. Olestra looks and tastes like real fat and it can withstand the high temperatures of frying.

Any side effects?

Because our bodies cannot digest or absorb olestra, some people experience a laxative effect (gas, abdominal cramping and loose stools). Symptoms vary according to the amount of olestra you consume, other foods you eat at the same time, and your individual response. The Food and Drug Administration (FDA) requires all olestra-containing foods to carry a warning label that alerts consumers to possible digestive effects.

Some researchers warn that olestra lowers blood levels of fat-soluble vitamins A, D, E and K and other cancer-fighting carotenoids (nutrients found in fruits and vegetables), such as beta-carotene. To offset the loss of vitamins A, D, E and K, these vitamins are "added back" to foods made with olestra, but carotenoids are not. Researchers say that over time this effect could result in additional cases of cancer and other diseases if Olean products become a regular part of the American diet.

Look for the whole package — taste and nutrition.

Olean snack foods look and taste like the real thing—without the calories and fat. Sound too good to be true? Maybe. Healthy eating requires more than just cutting back on the fat you eat. Eating foods made with Olean will not cure unhealthy habits, like skipping breakfast or skimping on fruits and vegetables. These foods will not improve your health or guarantee that you lose weight. Snacks made with Olean are simply that — snacks. And most chips and crackers won't win any nutrition contests.

The bottom line...

It's up to you to decide about eating foods made with olestra. Whatever snacks you choose, be sure to eat them with "real food" — not in place of it.

The Lowdown on Label Lingo

 Last time you cruised down an aisle in the grocery store, did you notice the endless number of foods labeled "low-fat," "fat-free," "reduced-fat" and "lite"? What's the difference? Can you believe these claims? Thousands of products crowd the shelves of a typical grocery store, and new ones pop up daily. What can you do? If you feel overwhelmed when it comes to making healthy choices, you're not alone. Arm yourself with some handy information on food labels and you'll be selecting nutritious foods in no time.

Hop on Board for a Food Label Tour

Food labels contain a gold mine of information. You just need to know where to dig for it. Take a minute and grab any food package and hop on board for a private tour of the food label.

The first stop on our label tour features the **Ingredients List**. Here you'll find exactly what is in a food. Ingredients are listed by weight from most to least. In other words, those in the largest amounts appear early (near the top) on the list, followed in order by ingredients present in lesser amounts. Compare the labels of two fruit drinks and see what you can unearth by just looking at the ingredient lists.

Juice #1

Ingredients: Water, high fructose corn syrup and 2% or less of each of the following: concentrated orange juice, concentrated tangerine juice, concentrated lime juice, concentrated grapefruit juice.

Juice #2

Ingredients: Orange juice, water.

Did you discover that ounce per ounce, juice #2 contains more juice than water or sugar (high fructose corn syrup)?

Our second stop focuses on the **Nutrition Facts** section. Here you can eyeball information on serving size, calories, and major nutrients such as fat, cholesterol, sodium, carbohydrates, protein, and various vitamins and minerals. Start by looking at the serving size listed. Is your serving the same size as the one on the label? If you eat double the serving size listed, you need to double the nutrient and calorie values. If you eat one-half the serving size shown, cut the nutrient and calorie values in half. Take a pit stop and check the label on page 101 for more specific information on serving size, calories and major nutrients.

The final stop on our label tour focuses on the **Nutrient Claims** found on food packages. As of 1994, the federal government regulates these claims. You can now trust the following key words when you see them appear on a food package.

KEY WORDS	WHAT THEY MEAN
Fat Free	Less than 0.5 grams of fat per serving.
Low Fat	3 grams of fat (or less) per serving.
Low in Saturated Fat	1 gram saturated fat (or less) per serving.
Lean	Less than 10 grams of fat, 4 grams of saturated fat and 95 milligrams of cholesterol per serving.
Extra Lean	Less than 5 grams of fat, 2 grams of saturated fat and 95 milligrams of cholesterol per serving.
Light or Lite	One-third fewer calories or 50% less fat per serving of original product.
Reduced, Less, Lower, Fewer	Food must have at least 25% less of the nutrient than the food it's being compared to.
Cholesterol Free	Less than 2 milligrams of cholesterol and 2 grams (or less) of saturated fat per serving. (This does not necessarily mean it's low in fat or calories.)
Percent Fat Free	May be used only on foods that are low-fat or fat-free to begin with. It is a reflection of the amount of the food's weight that is fat-free and is not the same as the percent of calories from fat. For example, a food labeled 95% fat-free (or 5% fat by weight) may actually contribute 35% of its calories from fat.
Low Sodium	140 milligrams of sodium (or less) per serving.
Sugar Free	Less than 0.5 grams of sugar per serving.
High Fiber	5 grams of fiber (or more) per serving.
Good Source of Fiber	2.5 to 4.9 grams of fiber per serving.

Serving Size
Always check the serving size. You may eat more or less than one serving; adjust the numbers accordingly. Keep in mind that the labeled serving size is not a recommended portion size.

Calories
Shows total calories (from fats, carbohydrates and proteins) in one serving.

Total Fat
Lists the total fat contained in one serving (includes monounsaturated, polyunsaturated and saturated fats). All fats listed are rounded off to the nearest .5 gram.

Saturated Fat
This is one of the several fats that constitute **Total Fat**. It's most responsible for raising blood cholesterol levels. Less than 10% of total calories should come from saturated fat.

Cholesterol
Not as significant as saturated fat, dietary cholesterol can also raise blood cholesterol levels. Eat less than 300 mg per day (less than 200 mg if you have high blood cholesterol levels).

Vitamins & Minerals
Your goal is 100% of each for the day, provided by a combination of healthy foods. One food can't do it all!

Calories from Fat
This helps you see how fatty a food is. You can calculate % fat as follows:

(Calories from Fat ÷ Total Calories) x 100

Example: (150 Calories from Fat ÷ 330 Total Calories) x 100 = 45% Calories from Fat

% Daily Value
This value shows how a food fits into the overall daily diet. Labels use a 2,000 calorie diet as a standard. Note: If a food has 20% or more of the Daily Value, it's considered a "significant" source of the nutrient. A "low" source would be less than 5%.

Sodium
No more than 2,400 mg a day is recommended for healthy adults.

Total Carbohydrate
This total includes several carbohydrate sources: complex carbohydrates (e.g. grains), sugars and dietary fiber.

Fiber: Foods containing 2.5 grams or more are good sources of fiber.

Sugars: This number isn't very precise; it includes naturally occurring fruit and milk sugars.

Tip: 1 teaspoon sugar = 4 grams of carbohydrate.

Nutrition Facts
Serving Size 1 cup (225g)
Servings Per Container 2½

Amount Per Serving

Calories 330   Calories from Fat 150

% Daily Value*

Total Fat 17g	**26%**
Saturated Fat 6g	**30%**
Cholesterol 30mg	**10%**
Sodium 940mg	**39%**
Total Carbohydrate 31g	**10%**
Dietary Fiber 2g	**8%**
Sugars 6g	
Protein 14g	

Vitamin A	2%	Vitamin C	0%
Calcium	30%	Iron	2%

Percent Daily Values are based on a 2,000 calorie diet. Your daily values may be higher or lower depending on your calorie needs:

		Calories	2,000	2,500
Total Fat	Less than		65g	80g
Sat Fat	Less than		20g	25g
Cholesterol	Less than		300mg	300mg
Sodium	Less than		2,400mg	2,400mg
Total Carbohydrate			300g	375g
Fiber			25g	30g

Calories per gram:
Fat 9 • Carbohydrate 4 • Protein 4

Take a Closer Look at the Labels on Meat — What Do the Numbers Really Mean?

You've seen the claims — ground beef labeled extra-lean or only 15 percent fat. Sounds great, but it doesn't mean what you think. In this case, ground beef is 15 percent fat by weight, not by calories. Here's the real scoop. A gram of fat contributes nine calories whereas a gram of protein or carbohydrate contributes only four. A three-ounce hamburger made with extra-lean ground beef contains 17 grams of fat and 250 calories, which means 61% of its calories come from fat!

Take a look at how the numbers work:

- Convert fat grams into fat calories: 17 grams of fat x 9 calories per gram = 153 fat calories.

- Divide the fat calories (153) by the total calories (250) and multiply by 100 to obtain the percent of calories from fat.

To select the leanest meats possible, read the labels and look at the total grams of fat per serving.

The Bottom Line

The foods you eat should taste good and give you the nutrients you need. Use food labels to help you make smart choices in matters of taste and nutrition.

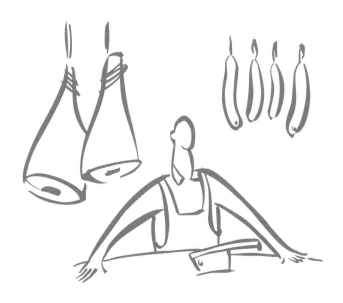

My S.M.A.R.T. Plans for this Week

Stop and take a few minutes to set up S.M.A.R.T. fitness and food plans for yourself this week. They may be the same or different than last week's plans.

S.M.A.R.T. FITNESS PLAN	S.M.A.R.T. FOOD PLAN
Specific What activity(s) will I do? Time of day? (a.m. or p.m.)	**S**pecific What will I work on?
Measurable How many days will I exercise? Which days will I exercise? How many minutes will I do it for?	**M**easurable How many days will I do it for? Which days will I target? (weekdays, weekends)
Achievable Is this plan realistic? Reasonable?	**A**chievable Is this plan realistic? Reasonable?
Relevant Is this an activity I enjoy? Can I make it a priority this week?	**R**elevant Will changing this eating habit make a difference in my health?
Trackable Where will I record my activity?	**T**rackable How will I monitor this behavior?

Skill Practice: Week Four

 Turn your new skills into new habits by concentrating your efforts on the following activities this week.

1. **Keep records** —Keep track of your eating habits using one of the following methods.

   ☐ Record food and fat content. To determine % calories from fat, record calories as well. (See suggestion.)

   ☐ Record food only.

   ☐ Record food and hunger/fullness cues.

   ☐ Use the Food Pyramid for a nutrition check. (See Appendix.)

   ☐ Record food and calories.

   ☐ My own tracking system

   (specify): _____

   Suggestion: Record everything that you eat and drink in your FOOD & ACTIVITY JOURNAL. Track your fat intake using food labels and the CALORIE & FAT COUNTER.

2. **S.M.A.R.T. plans** — Follow the fitness and food plans you made for yourself this week.

3. **Check food labels** — Take five minutes this week to check out the food labels on products located in your cupboard or in your grocery store. Compare the serving size to the amount you actually eat.

> *Reminder:* Don't forget to record your fitness activities in your FOOD & ACTIVITY JOURNAL.

FOOD & ACTIVITY JOURNAL

Date:_____

Day: M Tu W Th F Sat Sun

Fitness Activity:

TIME	FEELINGS CHECK	H/F SCALE*	FOOD & DRINK	AMOUNT	CALORIES	FAT (grams)	H/F SCALE*
					Total:	Total:	

*Rate your hunger/fullness on a scale from 0–10: 0 = Empty, 5 = Just Right, 10 = Stuffed

FOOD & ACTIVITY JOURNAL

Date:_____

Day: M   Tu   W   Th   F   Sat   Sun

Fitness Activity:

TIME	FEELINGS CHECK	H/F SCALE*	FOOD & DRINK	AMOUNT	CALORIES	FAT (grams)	H/F SCALE*
					Total:	Total:	

*Rate your hunger/fullness on a scale from 0–10: 0 = Empty, 5 = Just Right, 10 = Stuffed

FOOD & ACTIVITY JOURNAL

Date:_____

Day: M   Tu   W   Th   F   Sat   Sun

Fitness Activity:

TIME	FEELINGS CHECK	H/F SCALE*	FOOD & DRINK	AMOUNT	CALORIES	FAT (grams)	H/F SCALE*
					Total:	Total:	

*Rate your hunger/fullness on a scale from 0–10: 0 = Empty, 5 = Just Right, 10 = Stuffed

FOOD & ACTIVITY JOURNAL

Date:_____

Day: M   Tu   W   Th   F   Sat   Sun

Fitness Activity:

TIME	FEELINGS CHECK	H/F SCALE*	FOOD & DRINK	AMOUNT	CALORIES	FAT (grams)	H/F SCALE*
						Total:	Total:

*Rate your hunger/fullness on a scale from 0–10: 0 = Empty, 5 = Just Right, 10 = Stuffed

FOOD & ACTIVITY JOURNAL

Date:_____

Fitness Activity:	

Day: M   Tu   W   Th   F   Sat   Sun

TIME	FEELINGS CHECK	H/F SCALE*	FOOD & DRINK	AMOUNT	CALORIES	FAT (grams)	H/F SCALE*
					Total:	Total:	

*Rate your hunger/fullness on a scale from 0–10: 0 = Empty, 5 = Just Right, 10 = Stuffed

FOOD & ACTIVITY JOURNAL

Date:_____

Day: M   Tu   W   Th   F   Sat   Sun

Fitness Activity:	

TIME	FEELINGS CHECK	H/F SCALE*	FOOD & DRINK	AMOUNT	CALORIES	FAT (grams)	H/F SCALE*
					Total:	Total:	

*Rate your hunger/fullness on a scale from 0–10: 0 = Empty, 5 = Just Right, 10 = Stuffed

FOOD & ACTIVITY JOURNAL

Date:_____

Day: M   Tu   W   Th   F   Sat   Sun

Fitness Activity:_____

TIME	FEELINGS CHECK	H/F SCALE*	FOOD & DRINK	AMOUNT	CALORIES	FAT (grams)	H/F SCALE*
					Total:	Total:	

*Rate your hunger/fullness on a scale from 0–10: 0 = Empty, 5 = Just Right, 10 = Stuffed

Stay on Target

Do what you can, with what you have, where you are . . .
                                                —*Theodore Roosevelt*

Beware the "all or nothing" thinking trap when making healthy choices. It's easy to fall into this way of thinking, especially if you've ever been a "regular" on the dieting scene. Diets promote black and white thinking with lists of "good" and "bad" foods. The idea is to make progress, not to be perfect. Don't declare any foods forbidden or off limits; just watch the amounts you eat. If your passion is chocolate fudge ice cream, go ahead and savor a scoop occasionally. It won't matter, if you stay active and eat sensibly most of the time. Remember the 80/20 rule? Strive to make wise choices 80% of the time and go easy on yourself the other 20% of the time.

This Week You Will:

- Reflect over the previous week, noting insights and accomplishments.
- Check the progress you've made after one month.
- Identify factors that affect your metabolism, and recognize genetic influences.
- Explore the features of four different eating styles.
- Motivate yourself to keep moving with tips on physical activity.
- Design a personal S.M.A.R.T. plan for food and fitness.

Reflections

Reflect on your FOOD & ACTIVITY JOURNAL

Last week's suggestion was to track fat in your FOOD & ACTIVITY JOURNAL. If you did this activity, what did you learn? What changes, if any, do you plan to make with your fat budgeting?

Reflect on your S.M.A.R.T. plans

How did these plans work for you? Do you plan to use them again, throw them out or fine-tune them?

Other observations from last week

What worked well for you? What didn't work?

Facts of Life: Measuring Your Progress II

 You are now halfway through the *Smart CHOICES* program, past the honeymoon stage and into the realm of making lifestyle changes. Progress has many faces. Losing weight is only one reward that comes from eating healthier, being more active and gaining support for a new lifestyle. You still have work to do, but you may be surprised at how far you've come. Take a minute to review this list of progress indicators and check off the ones you have experienced since starting this program.

Healthier Eating Habits:

❑ I eat more fruits and vegetables.

❑ I eat more complex carbohydrates, such as whole grains and dried beans (legumes).

❑ I make lower-fat food choices.

❑ I plan ahead more often regarding meals and snacks.

❑ I eat smaller amounts.

Better Emotional Health:

❑ I pay more attention to my body's hunger/fullness signals (eat when hungry, stop before feeling stuffed).

❑ I no longer try to rigidly control my food by dieting.

❑ My attitude toward my body has improved (more respectful and accepting).

❑ I feel more at peace with food and the role it plays in my life.

❑ I am less critical of myself (less negative self-talk).

❑ I feel more capable of achieving and maintaining a healthier weight.

❑ I notice less emotional eating (I use food less often as a coping mechanism).

❑ I ask for support more often.

❑ I am more assertive in turning down food when I'm not hungry.

Improved Physical Health:

☐ I am more physically active on a regular basis.

☐ I've lost inches (body fat).

☐ I can climb stairs or carry packages more easily without getting short of breath.

☐ My clothes fit more comfortably.

☐ I am able to participate more fully in fun physical activities (such as hiking with the family).

☐ I have more energy throughout the day (fewer highs and lows).

☐ I move with greater ease.

Improved Medical Status:

☐ My blood sugars are under better control (improved diabetes control).

☐ My blood pressure is lower.

☐ My total cholesterol and/or LDL cholesterol level is lower.

☐ I am able to take less medication for a chronic health problem or illness.

Other Changes:

☐ _____

☐ _____

☐ _____

Reminder: Grab a tape measure and recheck the body measurements you took in Week One. Turn to page 14 and record your measurements.

Your Metabolism: Put It in Gear

 Wouldn't it be great to eat all you want and never gain an ounce? But your body has a built-in survival mechanism that works more efficiently than that. Any excess calories that you don't use or burn up, you store as body fat. In other words, body fat is essentially stored energy. In the days of "feast and famine," it was a benefit to have some extra stored energy on hand. Today we live in an era of "feast and feast" and we no longer depend on excess body fat for survival.

Metabolism 101	
Metabolism =	Rate at which you burn calories.
Muscle mass =	Portion of your body that burns calories (is metabolically active). Use it or lose it. If you don't use your muscle through physical activity, you will lose it over time.
Body fat =	Portion of your body that stores energy and takes up space, but doesn't burn any calories.
Weight loss goal =	Lose body fat while retaining as much muscle as possible.

Factors That Affect Your Metabolism

Many factors affect your metabolism. Some you can change, others you have no control over.

You CAN NOT control . . .

Heredity Your genetic makeup affects your body shape and size, as well as your ability to burn calories. You may be genetically programmed, for example, to be rounder in shape. Don't equate good health with being thin. Make the most of your body type within its genetic potential. You can't change your parents, but you can change the way you eat and how you move your body.

Age In general, as you age, you become less active. With physical inactivity, you lose muscle and gain fat. You can minimize this loss if you stay active as you age.

Gender Women naturally have more body fat and 10 to 20% less muscle than men do. Because of this difference in body composition (muscle vs. fat), men tend to burn more calories.

- Healthy body fat ranges for women: 17 to 24 percent.
- Healthy body fat ranges for men: 10 to 17 percent.

You CAN change or control . . .

Body Composition (Muscle vs. Fat)	Ounce for ounce, muscle burns more calories than body fat. The more muscle you have, the more calories you burn. The best way to build muscle is to do strength training exercises.
Calorie Intake	Fasting and very low-calorie diets cause a metabolic slowdown that shifts your body into a survival mode. Don't rely on these methods to lose weight and keep it off permanently. They always backfire. In the long run, yo-yo dieting causes you to need fewer calories to maintain the same weight.
Lifestyle	The amount you eat (calories in) and your activity level (calories out) directly impact your metabolism.

Ways To Rev Up Your Metabolism

Eat enough	Your metabolism slows if you don't eat ENOUGH calories. Experts recommend not dropping below 1200 to 1400 calories a day.
Be active	Physical activity boosts your metabolism in these ways: **Aerobic exercise** — you burn calories during exercise and for a short time afterwards. **Strength training** — resistance training (with weights, elastic bands or even soup cans) builds muscle. The more muscle you have, the more calories you burn.

Weight Loss: Is it Fat or Muscle?

When it comes to losing weight, the scale doesn't tell you whether you've lost fat, muscle or water. Keep in mind that losing weight always involves some loss of fat and muscle. Your goal should be to increase the amount of fat you lose while sparing the loss of muscle. The only way to do that — exercise while you are losing weight. These numbers tell the story:

	% Weight Loss That Is Muscle Mass	% Weight Loss That Is Fat
Reducing Calories + No Exercise	25 %	75 %
Reducing Calories + Exercise	5 %	95 %

Reference: B. Marks & J. Rippe, Sports Medicine, 22, 5 (1996), 273-281.

Eating in Style?

 Your eating style affects your energy level, the amount you eat, your food choices and ultimately your weight. Up to this point, you've focused on "what to eat" as part of a healthy diet. Now take a look at how the timing and distribution of your calories affect your efforts to lose pounds and maintain a healthy weight.

Make the Most of When You Eat

Do you eat most of your calories during the day or after the sun goes down? Take a look at the four eating patterns shown below. How does your eating style compare?

Meal & Snack Distribution:

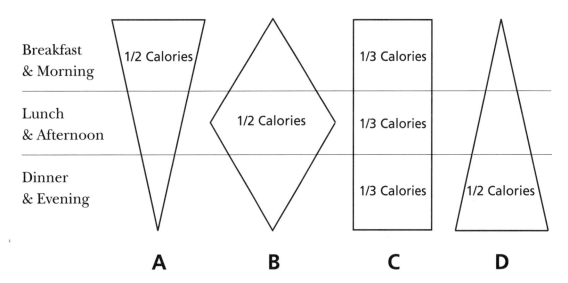

Pattern A—Breakfast stars as the main meal of the day. You eat a much smaller lunch and dinner by comparison. This rare eating pattern may suit a farmer who expends lots of energy in the early hours of the day.

Pattern B— You sandwich a midday calorie-rich meal between light breakfast and dinner meals. Many European countries favor this eating pattern.

Pattern C—You evenly distribute your food (and calories) among meals and snacks throughout the day. This eating pattern promotes a consistent energy level throughout the day.

Pattern D—You routinely skip breakfast and eat relatively small amounts during the day. Once you begin eating at dinner time, you continue throughout the evening. This style promotes a "feast or famine" pattern of eating.

In the old days, when the United States was a predominantly agricultural nation, Patterns A and B worked well for hard-working farmers who rose at the crack of dawn. Along with Pattern C, these eating patterns provide sufficient calories throughout the entire day. In other words, you have plenty of energy to get your chores done. By contrast, if you follow Pattern D—undereat during the day and overeat at night—you sabotage your energy level as well as your waistline.

Don't look for an energy boost from a "feast or famine" eating style. When you starve yourself during the day, you deprive your body of energy just when it needs it the most. You also set yourself up to overeat. When you feel ravenous late in the day, it's easy to ignore the "I'm full" signal once you start eating. It's also not surprising you lack an appetite for breakfast if you stuff yourself the night before.

Overeating in the evening may be due to emotional triggers. Be sensitive to your feelings and emotions at these times. Are you eating out of boredom, to reward yourself, or to numb how you feel? Pay attention to your feelings and check in with your hunger/fullness signals.

Analyze Your Eating Style

Take five minutes and analyze your eating style. Grab a FOOD & ACTIVITY JOURNAL (one complete day) and add up the calories for each of these time periods.

- Breakfast & a.m. calories = _____

- Lunch & afternoon calories = _____

- Dinner & p.m. calories = _____

Which pattern is your eating style (Pattern A, B, C, D)?

What, if any, changes could you make to your eating style?

Grazing vs. Three Squares

Some people eat "three squares" a day while others graze or nibble throughout the day. Frequent mini-meals or grazing can be an effective way to meet your nutritional needs. If you nibble constantly, however, and never let yourself become hungry, you may override your body's need for food. You want to balance the calories in meals and snacks with your body's need for energy. Pay attention to the hunger and fullness signals your body sends and plan your meals and snacks accordingly. For example, maybe you are a "1" (starved) on the HUNGER/FULLNESS SCALE at 11:00 a.m. and your lunch break doesn't come until noon. What should you do? Plan ahead and keep healthy snacks, such as pretzels or low-fat crackers, in your desk drawer to satisfy hunger pangs before they get out of control.

Grazing Styles

What do horses, sheep, goats, cows and people have in common? We all like to graze! Take a look at the grazing styles of these animals. How do you compare?

Horse　　Eats like a horse, has a "healthy appetite."

　　　　　　Pitfall: Beware of overeating when you graze.

Sheep　　Eats what everybody else does. Goes along with the herd, gives in to temptations.

　　　　　　Pitfall: Beware of succumbing to peer pressure, eating because "it's there and everyone else is eating."

Goat　　Eats garbage and "junk."

　　　　　　Pitfall: Beware of eating foods with little or no nutritional value.

Cow　　Eats steadily and consistently all day. Chooses high fiber foods, chews slowly.

　　　　　　Lesson: Eat like a cow!

Getting Physical: Tips for Exercise

You Set the Pace

Honor where you are right now. If you've been inactive, you'll want to start slow and gradually increase your activity. Pay attention to your body and go at a pace that feels right for you.

To Burn Fat, Get Moving

You burn fat and calories every time you move. It doesn't have to be "non-stop continuous, get-your-heart-rate-up" movement in order to burn calories, although these types of activity do wonders for your heart, lungs and endurance. Here's the bottom line — ANY type of physical activity burns fat and calories. So get moving! Park your car farther from the store, take the stairs instead of the elevator, walk into the bank instead of using the drive-up window, and retire your remote control. These may sound like little things, but they add up in the big picture.

How to Burn More Fat

The more you move, the more calories you burn and the faster you'll lose weight. If you're just starting out, slow down so that you can exercise for a longer period of time before you tire out. You'll burn more calories this way than if you work so hard that you quit after a few minutes. However, the higher your level of fitness, the harder and longer you can exercise without getting tired.

No Best Time

There is no "best time" to exercise. If you are a morning person, work out in the morning. If you're up with the owls, exercise at night. If you're short on time, spread your exercise throughout the day. For example, you will burn calories just as effectively in two 15-minute sessions as one 30-minute session.

Set a Fitness Goal

As you begin a fitness program, ask yourself: "Where do I want to be six months from now?" Your personal fitness goals will guide you in selecting an activity and setting up a weekly schedule.

Examples of personal fitness goals:

- I want to have more energy and more stamina. I will choose an aerobic activity, like brisk walking, to build my endurance.

- I want to be able to get out of a chair without assistance. I'll work on strengthening the muscles in my arms and legs.

- I want to be able to run three days a week for thirty minutes at a time without stopping. I will work on a walk-jog plan three days a week until I build up to a run.

My personal fitness goal: _____

_____

Remember that when it comes to fitness, any activity is better than none at all!

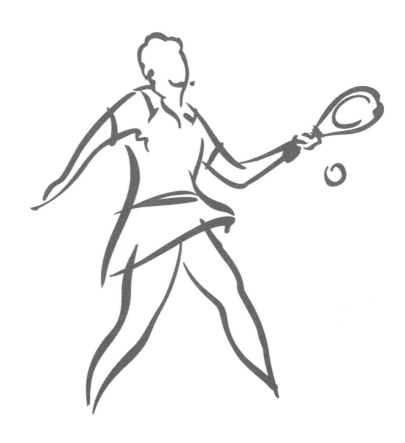

My S.M.A.R.T. Plans for this Week

Stop and take a few minutes to set up S.M.A.R.T. fitness and food plans for yourself this week. They may be the same or different than last week's plans.

S.M.A.R.T. FITNESS PLAN	S.M.A.R.T. FOOD PLAN
Specific What activity(s) will I do?	Specific What will I work on?
Time of day? (a.m. or p.m.)	
Measurable How many days will I exercise?	Measurable How many days will I do it for?
Which days will I exercise?	Which days will I target? (weekdays, weekends)
How many minutes will I do it for?	
Achievable Is this plan realistic? Reasonable?	Achievable Is this plan realistic? Reasonable?
Relevant Is this an activity I enjoy?	Relevant Will changing this eating habit make a difference in my health?
Can I make it a priority this week?	
Trackable Where will I record my activity?	Trackable How will I monitor this behavior?

Skill Practice: Week Five

 Focus on the following activities as you continue to learn about what works best for you in achieving a healthier lifestyle.

1. **Keep records** — Keep track of your eating habits using one of the following methods. You decide what to monitor this week.

   ☐ Record food only.

   ☐ Record food and hunger/fullness cues.

   ☐ Use the Food Pyramid for a nutrition check. (See Appendix.)

   ☐ Record food and calories.

   ☐ Record food and fat grams.

   ☐ My own tracking system

   (specify): _____

2. **S.M.A.R.T. plans** — Follow the fitness and food plans you made for yourself this week.

3. **Recheck your body measurements** — Grab a tape measure and recheck your measurements. Record your findings on page 14.

Reminder. Don't forget to record your fitness activities in your FOOD & ACTIVITY JOURNAL.

FOOD & ACTIVITY JOURNAL

Date:_____

Day: M   Tu   W   Th   F   Sat   Sun

Fitness
Activity:

TIME	FEELINGS CHECK	H/F SCALE*	FOOD & DRINK	AMOUNT	CALORIES	FAT (grams)	H/F SCALE*
					Total:	Total:	

*Rate your hunger/fullness on a scale from 0–10: 0 = Empty, 5 = Just Right, 10 = Stuffed

FOOD & ACTIVITY JOURNAL

Date:_____

Day: M   Tu   W   Th   F   Sat   Sun

Fitness Activity:	

TIME	FEELINGS CHECK	H/F SCALE*	FOOD & DRINK	AMOUNT	CALORIES	FAT (grams)	H/F SCALE*
					Total:	Total:	

*Rate your hunger/fullness on a scale from 0–10: 0 = Empty, 5 = Just Right, 10 = Stuffed

FOOD & ACTIVITY JOURNAL

Date:_____

Day: M   Tu   W   Th   F   Sat   Sun

Fitness
Activity:

TIME	FEELINGS CHECK	H/F SCALE*	FOOD & DRINK	AMOUNT	CALORIES	FAT (grams)	H/F SCALE*
					Total:	Total:	

*Rate your hunger/fullness on a scale from 0–10: 0 = Empty, 5 = Just Right, 10 = Stuffed

FOOD & ACTIVITY JOURNAL

Date:_____

Day: M   Tu   W   Th   F   Sat   Sun

Fitness Activity:

TIME	FEELINGS CHECK	H/F SCALE*	FOOD & DRINK	AMOUNT	CALORIES	FAT (grams)	H/F SCALE*
					Total:	Total:	

*Rate your hunger/fullness on a scale from 0–10: 0 = Empty, 5 = Just Right, 10 = Stuffed

FOOD & ACTIVITY JOURNAL

Date:_____

Day: M   Tu   W   Th   F   Sat   Sun

Fitness Activity:

TIME	FEELINGS CHECK	H/F SCALE*	FOOD & DRINK	AMOUNT	CALORIES	FAT (grams)	H/F SCALE*
					Total:	Total:	

*Rate your hunger/fullness on a scale from 0–10: 0 = Empty, 5 = Just Right, 10 = Stuffed

FOOD & ACTIVITY JOURNAL

Date:_____

Day: M   Tu   W   Th   F   Sat   Sun

Fitness Activity:

TIME	FEELINGS CHECK	H/F SCALE*	FOOD & DRINK	AMOUNT	CALORIES	FAT (grams)	H/F SCALE*
					Total:	Total:	

*Rate your hunger/fullness on a scale from 0–10: 0 = Empty, 5 = Just Right, 10 = Stuffed

FOOD & ACTIVITY JOURNAL

Date:_____

Day: M   Tu   W   Th   F   Sat   Sun

Fitness Activity:

TIME	FEELINGS CHECK	H/F SCALE*	FOOD & DRINK	AMOUNT	CALORIES	FAT (grams)	H/F SCALE*
					Total:	Total:	

*Rate your hunger/fullness on a scale from 0–10: 0 = Empty, 5 = Just Right, 10 = Stuffed

Week

6

Feed Your Soul

I haven't failed, I've found 10,000 ways that don't work . . .

—*Benjamin Franklin*

A slip is just a slip and nothing more. If you feel that you've had a "bad" day or week, relax and accept it for what it really is — a day or week when healthful choices slipped down on your list of priorities. It's easy to be thrown off track. An illness, house guests, business travel or a vacation can derail your healthy intentions. Setbacks are only temporary. After you acknowledge a slip for what it is, reflect back on the skills and techniques that helped you in the past. Immediately begin to use these tools to get back on track.

> ## This Week You Will:
>
> - Reflect over the previous week, noting insights and accomplishments.
> - Reinforce the connection between food and feelings.
> - Concentrate on eating for health and enjoyment.
> - Refresh your motivation to stick with your exercise plan.
> - Design a personal S.M.A.R.T. plan for food and fitness.

Reflections

Reflect on your FOOD & ACTIVITY JOURNAL

Last week you decided which aspect(s) of your daily eating habits to monitor. What did you learn from this activity?

Reflect on your S.M.A.R.T. plans

How did these plans work for you? Do you plan to use them again, throw them out or fine-tune them?

Other observations from last week

What worked well for you? What didn't work?

Make the Connection: Food and Your Feelings

 You have a bad day at the office.

You get stuck in a two-hour traffic jam and arrive late for a family celebration.

The kids get on your nerves and you explode.

Situations like these provoke feelings or emotions that can send you running straight for the nearest cookie jar. Most people comfort themselves with food at one time or another. Turning to food occasionally to soothe your feelings is not a problem. However, if you routinely use food to stifle rather than deal with your emotions, you sabotage your efforts to lose pounds or maintain a healthy weight.

Many people believe they can simply "will" themselves to stop overeating. Unfortunately, this usually doesn't work for very long. If your emotional needs go unmet because you don't have the skills to cope with or resolve unpleasant feelings, then you'll most likely return to food. To curb emotional eating, you need to do three things:

- Become more aware of your feelings.
- Recognize the unmet emotional needs that are signaled by these feelings.
- Learn how to meet your emotional needs more effectively without relying on food.

You can learn these skills. It just takes time and practice.

Styles of Emotional Eating

Emotional eating typically appears in one of two forms — binge eating or constant grazing. Do you recognize these behaviors?

1. Characteristics of Binge Eating:
- Eating a large volume of food while feeling out of control.
- Eating food alone.
- Consuming food very quickly without tasting or enjoying it.
- Feeling distressed (disgusted, depressed, ashamed, etc.) after eating.

2. Characteristics of Constant Grazing:
- Eating frequently, even when not physically hungry.
- Eating out of boredom, loneliness or nervousness.

Note: Be aware that some of these eating behaviors may also be symptoms of depression. To explore this issue further, consult your physician or mental health counselor.

Emotional Eating: How to Regain Control

Take a look at the step-by-step process you can use to fill an emotional hunger without turning to food.

Step 1. Identify Your Feelings

Feelings or emotions express how we are doing on the inside. Our feelings provide valuable information and feedback. Most of us receive messages from our families and society about what we should and should not feel. You're probably familiar with some of these messages: women shouldn't be angry, men shouldn't cry, and adults should be able to handle their own problems without help.

Try not to think of feelings as simply being good or bad. It's healthy to experience both pleasant and unpleasant feelings. Strong feelings are powerful, though, and can be frightening. Sometimes they threaten to overwhelm us. Learning to experience feelings directly and "riding them out" is a valuable skill.

When you try to avoid expressing how you really feel, it's easy to turn to food for comfort or relief. Unfortunately, when you cope in this manner, you lose in two ways: you experience an increase in weight, and your emotional needs remain unmet. Getting in touch with your feelings can be hard work, but it's worth the effort. Listed below are some strategies to help you get started.

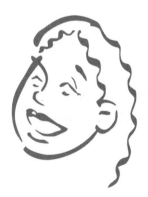

Stop and check on your feelings at various times throughout the day.

Feelings are valuable because they give you instant feedback about what's happening on the inside. Get in the habit of asking yourself, "What am I feeling right now?" If you find it difficult to identify your feelings, refer to the FEELING WORDS list on page 146. Using this list, choose the word(s) that most closely describes what you feel. Often you will feel several emotions at once. Be patient. If you've gotten out of the habit of recognizing or acknowledging your feelings, you will need to practice.

Learn to distinguish between a thought and a feeling.

Using the phrase I FEEL doesn't always mean that you are expressing a feeling. Either a feeling or a thought can follow this phrase.

When you share your feelings, you help others better understand your point of view by allowing them into your inner world. When you express only your thoughts and opinions, you run a greater risk of the listener feeling judged or on the defensive.

Example:

Thought: *I feel you should do more household chores.*

Feeling: *I feel **overwhelmed** by all the chores I do. I end up feeling **resentful** toward you about it, which I don't like.*

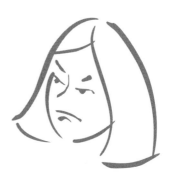

Differences Between a Thought and a Feeling

Thought	**Feeling**
• Often expressed as more than one word.	• Often expressed as one word.
• The phrases I FEEL YOU or I FEEL THAT…are always followed by a thought.	• You can substitute I AM for I FEEL in the sentence.
Examples of a thought:	*Examples of a feeling:*
I feel you don't care about me.	I feel sad. (I am sad.)
I feel that John will win the election this year.	I feel hopeful. (I am hopeful.)

Step 2. Use Feelings to Identify Your Needs

Feelings help you identify what you really need (other than food). Learning to translate your feelings into needs is a process that takes time. Be patient. You can use several different approaches to identify your needs, so choose what works for you.

How to Translate Your Feelings into Needs:

- **Use common sense or logic** — For example, if you feel lonely, you need to connect with someone; if you feel tired, you need to rest.

- **Trial and error** — Try something and see how well it meets your needs. Rate how satisfied you are with the results of what you have tried (1 = not satisfied, 3 = somewhat satisfied, 5 = very satisfied).

  Example: You feel sad.

  Option 1:   You eat and you feel worse. (rating = 1)

  Option 2:   You cry and feel better but still feel sad. (rating = 3)

  Option 3:   You cry, call a friend and share your sadness, and then make a plan to do something fun. This time you feel much better. (rating = 5)

- **Learn from others** — Seek help from people who seem good at meeting their needs in a healthy way. Ask them how they would handle a particular feeling to get what they need.

- **Keep it simple** — Express yourself as a young child would. Using a child's language, describe what you feel and what you need.

- **Keep a journal** — What are you feeling? What do you need? Even if you think you don't know the answer, start writing and see what answers come. There is no right or wrong way to keep a journal.

- **Identify familiar unpleasant feelings** — Make a list of unpleasant feelings that you frequently experience. Write down ways that might help you respond to these feelings and the needs they represent. If you get stuck, consider asking a supportive person for help and ideas. Add to this list, keep it accessible, and refer to it the next time these feelings come up.

Example:

FEELING	WAYS TO RESPOND TO FEELINGS/NEEDS WITHOUT FOOD
Sad	• Just be sad and let myself cry. • Write about it in a journal. • Talk to a supportive friend. • Do something physical (creates endorphins, the "feel good" chemicals in the brain). • Read or watch something fun or inspirational. • Do something that evokes sadness and helps me let it out (watch a sad movie, listen to sad music, etc.).
Lonely	• Seek out fun companionship. • Connect with nature (take a walk outdoors, plant flowers, etc.). • Play with a pet. • Make phone calls to friends.
Angry	• Write about it in a journal. • Write a "no-holds-barred" letter but don't send it. • Do something physical (walk, clean house, etc.). • Address the person or situation directly.
Anxious	• Identify negative self-talk and replace it with a reassuring, believable substitute. Instead of saying: I did a bad job with my presentation at work today! Change to: I am being overly hard on myself. It wasn't perfect, but it seemed to be well received.

Your turn! Using the chart below, take ten minutes and list at least three feelings that may lead you to overeat. Be sure you identify feelings and not thoughts (see Step 2). Write down possible ways you could respond to these feelings, and the needs they represent, without turning to food.

FEELINGS OR EMOTIONS	WAYS TO RESPOND TO FEELINGS/NEEDS WITHOUT FOOD
1.	
2.	
3.	

Step 3. Make Effective Requests: Communicating Your Feelings and Needs

When you identify your feelings and needs, you may also identify a request you need to make of someone else. Communicate your feelings using an **I FEEL** statement. Your listener will understand you better and be more sympathetic with your position if you express your feelings as part of your request. Watch out for I FEEL YOU… or I FEEL THAT… statements — they convey your thoughts, not your feelings.

Making a request doesn't guarantee that the other person will grant your request, but it does improve your chances of having your needs taken into account. Be aware of unrealistic expectations. For example, it may be unrealistic to expect your teenager to keep an immaculate room or your disorganized spouse to avoid misplacing things.

Note: There are times it makes sense to express needs but NOT feelings:

- With people who have been uncaring in response to your feelings in the past; for example, with anyone who tends to bully, criticize or manipulate you and would use your feelings to do so.

- Formal relationships where sharing the feelings behind your needs is inappropriate. For example, you have a colleague at work who is long-winded and rambles a lot. You feel irritated and frustrated at how much time you waste with this person. You need to limit the conversation. Expressing your irritation and frustration would not benefit either party.

Step 4. Identify Attitudes and Beliefs That Get in Your Way

Sometimes we act as our own worst enemies. Very often our own attitudes and beliefs set up the biggest barriers to meeting our needs. For example, when you say YES to a request when you want to say NO, you sacrifice your own needs in order to fulfill someone else's needs. These kinds of attitudes and beliefs can easily undermine your well-being and lead to emotional overeating.

Take a moment and check which attitudes you have experienced.

☐   I have to do it all perfectly.

☐   I can't take time to relax, be with friends, do fun things or rest. Too much work always needs to be done.

☐   It's not OK to say NO to another person's request or ask them to take care of their own needs.

☐   I've been hurt before, so it's not safe or worth it to risk trusting or depending on others.

☐   It's not OK to get angry, confused or otherwise experience a negative feeling.

     It's not OK to ask for support because:

     ☐   It burdens others.

     ☐   I should be able to handle it all myself.

     ☐   I would feel awful if I asked and was refused.

     It's not OK to put my own needs first; therefore, I never:

     ☐   Risk disappointing others in order to take care of myself.

     ☐   Spend time or money on myself.

     ☐   Do something just because it feels good.

More About the Connection Between Feelings and Overeating

If your feelings and emotions play a key role in influencing your weight, you may want to consider seeking further help in this area.

- Read more on the topic. For a list of books, refer to the Selected Resources section in the Appendix. Many of the recommended books contain activities and writings to help you understand behaviors and make changes.

- Join a support group.

- Seek help from a therapist who specializes in emotional eating issues.

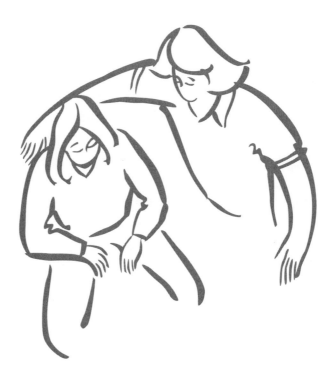

Emotional Eating: Taking Back Control

This week, or any time you find yourself fleeing to the cookie jar because of an unpleasant feeling or an emotionally charged situation, STOP and take ten minutes to complete this worksheet. You'll work through your feelings and needs and you will feel calmer. Before filling out your own worksheet, see the example on the following page.

EMOTIONAL EATING: TAKING BACK CONTROL WORKSHEET

Step 1. Identify Your Feelings

What are you feeling? It's possible to feel more than one emotion at a time. Write them all down. Use I FEEL statements.

I feel stressed out and overwhelmed because I have a big project due at work in one week.

Step 2. Use Feelings to Identify Your Needs

Your feelings help you identify what you need. Write down possible ways of meeting these needs without food. Note: If you have difficulty identifying your needs, refer to How to Translate Your Feelings into Needs in Step 2.

I need help! I need to delegate some of my responsibilities at work and ask my spouse for more support at home.

Step 3. Make Effective Requests: Communicate Your Feelings and Needs

After you identify your feelings and your needs, you may want to use this information to make a request. (In some cases, you may identify what you need from yourself as well as from others.) Communicate your feelings using an I FEEL statement.

To spouse: I feel overwhelmed with this big project due at work. I need more help around the house since I will be putting in extra hours at work. Would you please be in charge of dinner for the next week? I'll make dinners for the week following my project deadline.

To coworker: I feel overwhelmed with the big project due next week. I need some help. Would you be willing to take over my ordering responsibilities this week?

Step 4. Identify Attitudes and Beliefs That Get in the Way

Be alert to any attitudes that undermine your well-being. List any attitudes and beliefs that may become obstacles to getting your needs met.

I can do it all myself. I shouldn't impose on others by asking for their help.

It's not easy to identify your feelings and communicate your needs. Be patient with yourself while you learn. As with any other skill, you'll get better with practice.

Any time you experience an unpleasant feeling or an emotionally charged situation and you find yourself turning to food, STOP and take five to ten minutes to complete this worksheet. You'll work through your feelings and needs and you will feel calmer. Be patient. The more often you use this worksheet, the more skilled you will become at controlling your emotional eating. If you stumble with completing a step, refer back to the appropriate section of this chapter for help.

(For future use, a blank copy of this page is in the Appendix.)

EMOTIONAL EATING: TAKING BACK CONTROL WORKSHEET

Step 1. Identify Your Feelings

What are you feeling? It's possible to feel more than one emotion at a time. Write them all down. Use I FEEL statements.

Step 2. Use Feelings to Identify Your Needs

Your feelings will help you identify what you need. Write down possible ways of meeting these needs without food.

Step 3. Make Effective Requests: Communicate Your Feelings and Needs

After you identify your feelings and your needs, you may want to use this information to make a request. (In some cases, you may identify what you need from yourself as well as from others.) Communicate your feelings using an I FEEL statement.

Step 4. Identify Attitudes and Beliefs That Get in the Way

Be alert to any attitudes that undermine your well-being. List any attitudes and beliefs that may become obstacles to getting your needs met.

Feeling Words

HAPPY			
Levels of Intensity:			
Strong	Excited Jubilant	Thrilled Terrific	Joyful Loved	Ecstatic Enthusiastic
Medium	Proud Valued Amused	Cheerful Confident Delighted	Grateful Admired Optimistic	Accepted Appreciated Encouraged
Mild	Glad Peaceful	Good Satisfied	Pleased Hopeful	Content Fortunate

CONFUSED			
Strong	Bewildered Baffled	Trapped Constricted	Flustered Stagnant	Immobilized
Medium	Foggy Hesitant Perplexed	Doubtful Torn Puzzled	Ambivalent Troubled Awkward	Misunderstood Disorganized Distracted
Mild	Surprised Uncertain	Unsure Undecided	Bothered Unsettled	Uncomfortable

SAD			
Strong	Hopeless Miserable Crushed Wounded	Helpless Unwanted Worthless Dejected	Defeated Unloved Deserted Depressed	Devastated Sorrowful Hurt Rejected
Medium	Lonely Distant Guilty Inadequate	Resigned Isolated Abandoned Deprived	Ashamed Alienated Neglected Humiliated	Disappointed Upset Slighted Wasted
Mild	Sorry Deflated	Bad	Apathetic	Lost

ANGRY			
Strong	Abused Incensed Repulsed	Enraged Furious Betrayed	Hostile Hateful Exploited	Rebellious Outraged Mad
Medium	Offended Disgusted Smothered Aggravated	Irritated Annoyed Frustrated Controlled	Provoked Harassed Agitated Exasperated	Resentful Coerced Deceived Peeved
Mild	Uptight	Dismayed	Intolerant	Displeased

The Joy of Eating

 Eating occupies a significant part of life. The foods you eat should deliver the taste you want and the nutrition you need. This list of reminders will help you in your quest to balance taste and nutrition in the foods you choose.

Listen to your body—Eat when you are physically hungry, and stop when you feel satisfied. Never let yourself get too hungry; it sets you up for overeating.

Deprivation will get you nowhere—When you crave a certain food, stop and do a quick mental check. Ask yourself: "Do I really want this? Will I feel deprived if I don't have it?" If you answer "Yes," eat a reasonable portion and enjoy every bite of it. Avoid the temptation to nag yourself about your choice. Nagging just leads to guilty feelings and another serving.

Challenge the food police—Remind yourself that lists of "good" foods and "bad" foods do not exist. Eating should be a pleasurable, guilt-free experience based on internal cues of hunger and fullness, not external food plans or diets.

Plan your meals and snacks ahead of time—Stock your desk drawer, car and home with tasty foods that provide energy and other healthy benefits, such as dried apricots (vitamin A and fiber), string cheese (calcium and protein), and whole-grain crackers (carbohydrates and fiber). Balance a less healthy food with a nutritional powerhouse: a brownie with a glass of milk, for example. See Appendix for healthy meal and snack ideas.

Explore the fun side of food—Eat for enjoyment. Slow down and savor the aromas, textures and flavors that food brings to the table. Before you automatically reach for seconds, relax for a few minutes and check in with your feelings of hunger and fullness.

Clean Up Your Food Environment

Support your efforts to eat healthy by cleaning up your food environment. Keep problem foods out of the house. You know the ones — foods that tempt you from behind the refrigerator or cupboard doors, like chips, cookies, chocolate and ice cream. Consider it a problem food if you can't keep your hands off it.

You don't want to totally deprive yourself of these foods. On the other hand, if they end up in your house, before you know it they are in your mouth as well. How do you handle this dilemma? Use your skill power instead of willpower. If you crave a chocolate chip cookie, go to a bakery and buy one. Savor every bite and resist the urge to feel guilty. Just don't bring a dozen cookies home with you.

You need to accept the fact that you won't ever be able to eat whatever you want, whenever you want it, and still maintain a healthy weight. Developing your skill power allows you to enjoy these foods but in limited amounts. Having skill power will help you satisfy a craving for chips with a snack-size bag instead of the super size. Or, go out for a scoop of your favorite ice cream instead of bringing home a half gallon.

Exercise: How to Stay On Course

 Healthy eating and exercise go hand in hand. You're more likely to lose more weight and keep it off long-term if you exercise regularly. Set modest goals and stay motivated by incorporating the tips listed below.

Consistency Counts—Build exercise into your daily routine. It's more likely to become a habit if you set aside a specific time for it.

Spice It Up—Try a variety of activities to prevent boredom. Challenge yourself by trying a new sport, exercise class or piece of exercise equipment.

Plan Ahead—*If you exercise in the morning:* set out your exercise clothes and shoes the night before. If you prefer a cup of java before you start, set up the coffee pot too.

If you exercise after work: prepare your exercise bag the night before and set it next to the door. Exercise before going home from work. If you stop at home first, family members, the phone, the mail or the TV will likely derail you.

Smarten Up—Knowledge is power. Use it to fuel your motivation. Read fitness articles, magazines and books, or talk to a fitness specialist.

Take It Easy—Don't overdo it. Exercise at a pace that you could come back to tomorrow and repeat. Set reasonable goals for increases in intensity or duration.

Reward Yourself—When you fulfill your S.M.A.R.T. plans or feel you are making progress in the right direction, treat yourself to a movie, a book or magazine, or new workout clothes. Rewarding yourself for progress reinforces your new habit.

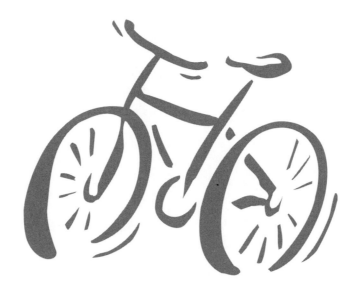

My S.M.A.R.T. Plans for this Week

Stop and take a few minutes to set up S.M.A.R.T. fitness and food plans for yourself this week. They may be the same or different than last week's plans.

S.M.A.R.T. FITNESS PLAN	S.M.A.R.T. FOOD PLAN
Specific What activity(s) will I do? Time of day? (a.m. or p.m.) **M**easurable How many days will I exercise? Which days will I exercise? How many minutes will I do it for? **A**chievable Is this plan realistic? Reasonable? **R**elevant Is this an activity I enjoy? Can I make it a priority this week? **T**rackable Where will I record my activity?	**S**pecific What will I work on? **M**easurable How many days will I do it for? Which days will I target? (weekdays, weekends) **A**chievable Is this plan realistic? Reasonable? **R**elevant Will changing this eating habit make a difference in my health? **T**rackable How will I monitor this behavior?

Skill Practice: Week Six

 Use these activities as an opportunity to further explore what works best for you in establishing healthy habits.

1. **Keep records** — Keep track of your eating habits using one of the following methods.

   ☐ Record your feelings before each meal or snack. (See suggestion.)

   ☐ Record food only.

   ☐ Record food and hunger/fullness cues.

   ☐ Use the Food Pyramid for a nutrition check. (See Appendix.)

   ☐ Record food and calories.

   ☐ Record food and fat grams.

   ☐ My own tracking system

       (specify): _____

   Suggestion: Check in with your feelings before each meal or snack. Record your observations in your FOOD & ACTIVITY JOURNAL. (If you need help identifying your feelings, use the FEELING WORDS listed on page 146.)

2. **Food/feeling connection** — To further explore the connection between your emotions and eating patterns, complete the EMOTIONAL EATING: TAKING BACK CONTROL WORKSHEET when an appropriate situation arises.

3. **S.M.A.R.T. plans** — Follow the fitness and food plans you made for yourself this week.

> *Reminder:* Don't forget to record your fitness activities in your FOOD & ACTIVITY JOURNAL.

FOOD & ACTIVITY JOURNAL

Date:_____

Day: M Tu W Th F Sat Sun

Fitness Activity:	

TIME	FEELINGS CHECK	H/F SCALE*	FOOD & DRINK	AMOUNT	CALORIES	FAT (grams)	H/F SCALE*
					Total:	Total:	

*Rate your hunger/fullness on a scale from 0–10: 0 = Empty, 5 = Just Right, 10 = Stuffed

FOOD & ACTIVITY JOURNAL

Date:_____

Day: M   Tu   W   Th   F   Sat   Sun

Fitness
Activity:

TIME	FEELINGS CHECK	H/F SCALE*	FOOD & DRINK	AMOUNT	CALORIES	FAT (grams)	H/F SCALE*
					Total:	Total:	

*Rate your hunger/fullness on a scale from 0–10: 0 = Empty, 5 = Just Right, 10 = Stuffed

FOOD & ACTIVITY JOURNAL

Date:_____

Day: M   Tu   W   Th   F   Sat   Sun

Fitness Activity:

TIME	FEELINGS CHECK	H/F SCALE*	FOOD & DRINK	AMOUNT	CALORIES	FAT (grams)	H/F SCALE*
					Total:	Total:	

*Rate your hunger/fullness on a scale from 0–10: 0 = Empty, 5 = Just Right, 10 = Stuffed

FOOD & ACTIVITY JOURNAL

Date:_____

Day: M   Tu   W   Th   F   Sat   Sun

Fitness Activity:

TIME	FEELINGS CHECK	H/F SCALE*	FOOD & DRINK	AMOUNT	CALORIES	FAT (grams)	H/F SCALE*
					Total:	Total:	

*Rate your hunger/fullness on a scale from 0–10: 0 = Empty, 5 = Just Right, 10 = Stuffed

FOOD & ACTIVITY JOURNAL

Date:_____

Day: M   Tu   W   Th   F   Sat   Sun

Fitness Activity:

TIME	FEELINGS CHECK	H/F SCALE*	FOOD & DRINK	AMOUNT	CALORIES	FAT (grams)	H/F SCALE*
					Total:	Total:	

*Rate your hunger/fullness on a scale from 0–10: 0 = Empty, 5 = Just Right, 10 = Stuffed

FOOD & ACTIVITY JOURNAL

Date:_____

Day: M   Tu   W   Th   F   Sat   Sun

Fitness Activity:	

TIME	FEELINGS CHECK	H/F SCALE*	FOOD & DRINK	AMOUNT	CALORIES	FAT (grams)	H/F SCALE*
					Total:	Total:	

*Rate your hunger/fullness on a scale from 0–10: 0 = Empty, 5 = Just Right, 10 = Stuffed

FOOD & ACTIVITY JOURNAL

Date:_____

Day: M   Tu   W   Th   F   Sat   Sun

Fitness Activity:

TIME	FEELINGS CHECK	H/F SCALE*	FOOD & DRINK	AMOUNT	CALORIES	FAT (grams)	H/F SCALE*
					Total:	Total:	

*Rate your hunger/fullness on a scale from 0–10: 0 = Empty, 5 = Just Right, 10 = Stuffed

Recipes for Success

If you find yourself reaching for food when you aren't hungry, stop and ask yourself: "What do I really want or need right now?" Perhaps you actually need to take a break and relax, talk to someone about a problem or get a hug from a supportive friend. Check in with your feelings for instant clues about how to best feed your "hunger."

> **This Week You Will:**
>
> - Reflect over the previous week, noting insights and accomplishments.
> - Restructure your thinking to turn negative internal conversations into positive "mental tapes."
> - Learn about healthy LEAN, LIGHT and LESS cooking techniques.
> - Discover simple solutions to rely on when navigating obstacles to fitness.
> - Design a personal S.M.A.R.T. plan for food and fitness.

Reflections

 ### Reflect on your FOOD & ACTIVITY JOURNAL

Which aspect(s) of your food intake/eating habits did you track? What did you learn from this activity?

Reflect on food/feeling connections

What did you learn from checking in with your feelings before you ate, or completing the EMOTIONAL EATING: TAKING BACK CONTROL worksheet?

Reflect on your S.M.A.R.T. plans

How did these plans work for you? Do you plan to use them again, throw them out or fine-tune them?

Other observations from last week

What worked well for you? What didn't work?

Self–Talk: Say the Right Thing

 You constantly talk to yourself throughout the day whether you are aware of it or not. This mental chit-chat or self-talk has the power to boost or squash your efforts to reach your goals. In fact, negative self-talk can turn you into your own worst enemy. It erodes your motivation and puts up barriers between you and a healthy lifestyle. On the other hand, positive self-talk can propel you toward your goals.

Think of your self-talk as "mental tapes" that stem from your beliefs, family upbringing, cultural background and life experiences. Listen to what you say to yourself. Do you tend to be positive and encouraging or negative and judgmental?

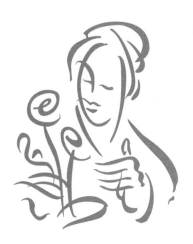

Self-Talk Examples

NEGATIVE SELF-TALK	POSITIVE SELF-TALK
I blew it!	*I had a setback but I know I can do it.*
I'll never be able to.	*I'll just do my best today.*
I'm not good enough.	*I don't have to be perfect to be lovable.*
I have no willpower.	*Food doesn't control me; I make the decisions about what, when and how much to eat.*
I shouldn't eat sweets. If I eat sweets, I'll never lose weight!	*It's OK to eat a sweet treat now and then. I won't gain weight from eating this one dessert. I'll try to eat it slowly and savor every bite.*

How Your Thoughts and Self-Talk Affect Your Behavior:

I think I can, I think I can . . . remember the "Little Engine That Could"? Your thoughts and how you talk to yourself affect the way you feel about yourself and ultimately your behavior. Take a look at how negative and positive self-talk influences the behavior and outcome of the following situation.

Situation: A coworker brings in two dozen freshly baked doughnuts and places them in the break room.

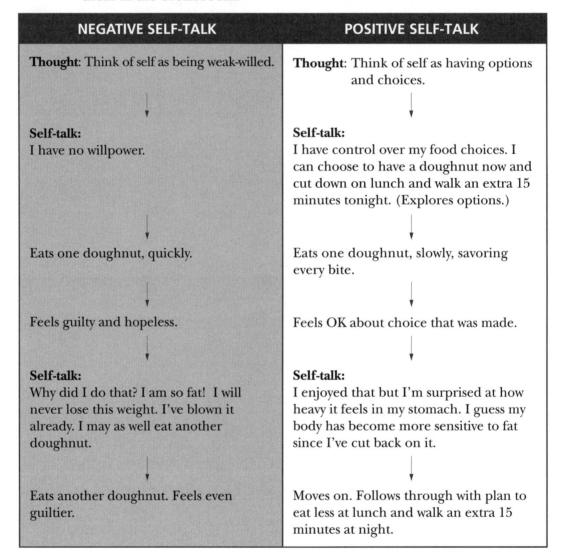

NEGATIVE SELF-TALK	POSITIVE SELF-TALK
Thought: Think of self as being weak-willed.	**Thought**: Think of self as having options and choices.
Self-talk: I have no willpower.	**Self-talk:** I have control over my food choices. I can choose to have a doughnut now and cut down on lunch and walk an extra 15 minutes tonight. (Explores options.)
Eats one doughnut, quickly.	Eats one doughnut, slowly, savoring every bite.
Feels guilty and hopeless.	Feels OK about choice that was made.
Self-talk: Why did I do that? I am so fat! I will never lose this weight. I've blown it already. I may as well eat another doughnut.	**Self-talk:** I enjoyed that but I'm surprised at how heavy it feels in my stomach. I guess my body has become more sensitive to fat since I've cut back on it.
Eats another doughnut. Feels even guiltier.	Moves on. Follows through with plan to eat less at lunch and walk an extra 15 minutes at night.

Tuning In to Self-Talk

Do you ever tune in to your internal conversations? Try it. If you feel unhappy, for example, check in with your self-talk. You may find it hard to maintain a positive self-image if you constantly beat yourself up mentally. Any time you feel depressed, anxious or guilty, check on your "mental tapes." What are you saying to yourself? Is your thinking based on reality? If not, what is the reality of the situation?

Confronting negative self-talk gives you the power to move forward with your plans for a healthier lifestyle. Irrational thinking often triggers negative self-talk. Try to counter negative self-talk with believable, positive (or at least neutral) statements. Many forms of distorted thinking exist, but the examples on the next page represent common themes that typically run through negative self-talk.

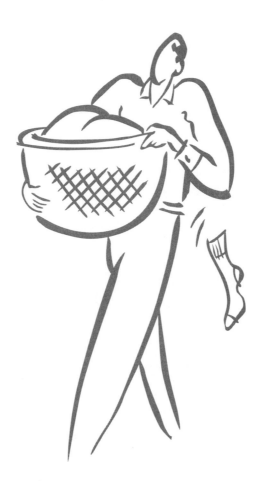

Going Down the Wrong Road

All-or-Nothing Self-Talk:

You see things as black and white, good or bad, either/or. No middle ground or shades of gray exist. You have to be perfect or you see yourself as a failure.

Example: *If I'm going to lose weight, I'll have to give up sweets and exercise daily until I reach my goal.*

Balanced Self-Talk: *I'll have to cut down on my sweets and be more active, but I can allow myself occasional desserts and occasional days without exercise.*

Filtering Self-Talk:

You notice all your faults and failures while ignoring your good points and successes.

Example: *I feel awful; I'm halfway through this program and I'm still not exercising daily (my original goal).*

Balanced Self-Talk: *I'm exercising three to four times a week on a regular basis; before this program I wasn't exercising at all. I can tell I'm getting in better shape. I'm still working on adding more days, but I'm already doing a good job!*

Overgeneralizing Self-Talk:

If something bad happens, you expect it to happen over and over again. You use words like always, never, all, every, none, no one, nobody, everyone and everybody in response to a situation.

Example: *I gained three pounds last week when I was sick; something always gets in the way. I'll never achieve my goal.*

Balanced Self-Talk: *Last week was a setback. Unplanned circumstances interfere sometimes, but most of the time I can continue on track. I know that in time I will reach my goal.*

Catastrophizing Self-Talk:

You anticipate a negative outcome and then act as if it were an established fact.

Example: *I gained two pounds last week. At this rate, I'll gain over 100 pounds this year.*

Balanced Self-Talk: *There is no reason to think this is the beginning of a long-term pattern. Weight fluctuations are normal. If I continue to practice healthy lifestyle choices, I'll continue to lose weight despite small fluctuations.*

Labeling Self-Talk:

You attach a label to yourself instead of simply describing the mistake.

Example: *I blew it at dinner. I'm a failure.*

Balanced Self-Talk: *It's OK not to be perfect. Just because I overate at one meal doesn't mean I will continue this pattern of eating.*

Egocentric Self-Talk:

You think that everything people do or say is some kind of reaction to you.

Example: *She didn't smile when she said good morning to me. What did I do to make her mad?*

Balanced Self-Talk: *There are many reasons she might not have smiled that have nothing to do with me. I'll watch how our next interaction goes. If she seems unfriendly, I can ask if it has anything to do with me.*

"Should" Self-Talk:

If shoulds don't happen, you feel let down.

Example: *I should have known better than to have a second helping.*

Balanced Self-Talk: *I am still learning to pay attention to my body's hunger/fullness signals. It takes practice and I'm getting better.*

Challenging Negative Self-Talk

The best way to counter negative self-talk is to catch yourself in the act. In this way, you can counter quickly with a balanced and positive (or at least neutral) statement. These statements must be believable. It may feel awkward or artificial at first. Hang in there, you'll get better with practice.

Next time you find yourself tripped up by irrational or negative thoughts, launch a counterattack by using one or more of the following balanced-thinking techniques.

- **Reality check.** Are your thoughts rational and/or realistic given the nature of the situation? Where's the evidence? If you feel terrible, examine the facts. Under close scrutiny, you'll often find your negative thoughts simply don't ring true. Uncertain whether your thoughts are based on fact or fiction? Get feedback from people you feel close to.

- **No put-downs.** Be careful not to label yourself negatively when you make a mistake. Separate who you are as a person from your behavior. Remind yourself that you don't need to be perfect to be lovable.

- **Speak in a gentle voice.** Refrain from yelling at yourself when you make a mistake. Instead, speak as you would to a good friend or young child, using a supportive and encouraging voice.

- **Watch out for "should" language.** Resist finger-wagging and scolding yourself. You can't move forward with a finger in your face.

- **Shades of gray.** Watch out for black and white thinking. Things in life are rarely "good" or "bad," "right" or "wrong." Try to view slip-ups objectively. You didn't blow it — you just chose a less healthy option in a particular situation. Your choice this time doesn't have any bearing on future decisions.

Learning to Counter Your Negative Self-Talk

Take five minutes and evaluate your negative internal conversations. Select two forms of distorted thinking from the preceding list that you tend to use. Write a typical example of the negative self-talk you would say to yourself. Then counter it with a positive, believable alternative.

NEGATIVE SELF-TALK	POSITIVE SELF-TALK
Example: All-or-nothing self-talk I will never be able to lose weight. I will always be fat. • •	**Counter to negative self-talk** Who said this would be easy? It took me years to gain this weight, it's not going to come off overnight. I don't want to give up now and waste my efforts. I can stick with it. • •

The way you talk to yourself is a habit, just like the way you choose foods. You can learn to switch to a more positive pattern of thinking. Don't like the tape that's playing? Pull it out and replace it with a new one. Like any new skill, it takes time and practice.

Countering Negative Self-Talk Worksheet

When you catch yourself slipping into negative self-talk this week, stop and take a minute to write it down. After recording it, take another minute to construct a balanced self-talk statement that counters your negative thought(s). Write these statements in the appropriate areas below.

NEGATIVE SELF-TALK	BALANCED SELF-TALK

Smart Cooking—Lean, Light and Less

 Fresh grilled salmon, hot crusty bread, a crispy salad with mixed greens, and oven-roasted potatoes with garlic and rosemary. Sound good? When you eat healthy foods, you don't have to do without or give up taste. Eating healthy means exploring a new world of foods, textures and flavors. It opens the door to a kitchen full of new seasonings, recipes and cooking methods.

Balancing taste and nutrition to achieve a healthier weight boils down to three main ingredients: the foods you purchase, cooking methods and how much you consume. You can learn to lower the fat and calories in your favorite foods with the three L's: lean, light and less.

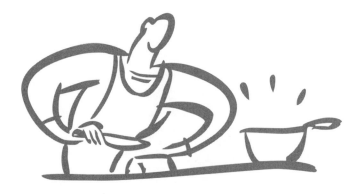

LEAN: Choose lighter or lower-fat versions of foods

Try different brands

Don't head straight for the shelves of fat-free products as you experiment with a lower-fat eating style. You'll most likely try a few, throw up your hands in disgust and return to your old fatty favorites. Fat-free products are not created equal. Just ask your taste buds. As with any product in the grocery store, some are tasty and some are downright unpalatable. You need to experiment and find products that suit your tastes. You may discover that fat-free cream cheese works great in your cheesecake recipe but not on your bagel. Or, you may enjoy the taste of skim milk from Joe's Grocery Store but dislike the brand from Fran's Grocery Store. Different brands taste different. It's simply a matter of trial and error to find products that will satisfy your taste buds.

Somewhere on the fat continuum between fat-free and mega-fat, you'll find a group of foods called "reduced" or "lower" fat. These foods tend to have 25 to 50 percent less fat than their regular counterparts. Since they retain some of their fat, however, reduced-fat foods still have the creamy taste and texture of regular products. Don't be fat phobic. Give these products a try. Your goal should be to cut down on the fat you eat, not totally eliminate it from your diet.

Label lingo

Fat-free, low fat, lean, reduced fat, less fat … these words scream at us from grocery shelves. The use of so many different terms can be confusing. Here's a quick review of what these label terms mean.

Fat Free	Less than 0.5 grams of fat per serving
Low Fat	3 grams of fat (or less) per serving
Low in Saturated Fat	1 gram of saturated fat (or less) per serving
Lean	Less than 10 grams of fat, 4 grams of saturated fat and 95 milligrams of cholesterol per serving
Extra Lean	Less than 5 grams of fat, 2 grams of saturated fat and 95 milligrams of cholesterol per serving
Reduced, Less, Lower, Fewer	Food must have at least 25% less of the nutrient than the food it's being compared to
Cholesterol Free	Less than 2 milligrams of cholesterol and 2 grams (or less) of saturated fat per serving. *Beware:* These foods are not necessarily low in fat or calories

Fat-free products

A fat-free label doesn't guarantee that a food is healthy or even lower in calories. For example, extra sugar often replaces the fat removed from cookies and baked goods. Though lower in fat, most fat-free brands contain almost as many calories as their regular counterparts. Misconceptions about fat-free foods lead many people to overindulge: It's fat-free, so have some more! This misguided attitude can lead to overeating and an expanded waistline.

There's more to food than just the fat

You're headed down the wrong road if you pass on salad at the dinner table because you dislike the taste of fat-free salad dressing. From a health standpoint, it makes more sense to have a salad with a little fat than miss out on an opportunity to consume vitamins, minerals, phytochemicals and fiber. You may find you eat even more veggies and salad if you keep a bottle of regular or reduced-fat salad dressing on hand.

Meat eaters: Indulge in leaner cuts but don't forget the pasta

Your heart, and your waistline, will benefit when you switch to eating leaner cuts of meat. Lean cuts (labeled round or loin) tend to be lower in fat, saturated fat and calories. When it comes time to fill your dinner plate, however, meat should not be the star attraction. That honor belongs to grains, bread, pasta and other complex carbohydrates located at the bottom of the Food Guide Pyramid. Keep meat servings small — about the size of a deck of cards.

Examples of LEAN food choices:

- Use nonfat or 1% versions of milk, yogurt and cottage cheese.

- Eat reduced-fat cheese in sandwiches (cheese with 6 grams of fat or less per ounce).

- Select sorbet instead of ice cream for dessert.

- Eat fish, skinless chicken, and dishes that feature beans and legumes instead of high-fat cuts of meat.

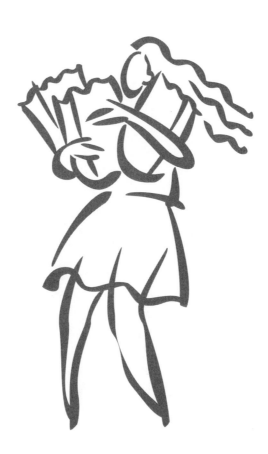

LIGHT: Prepare food the "light" way

When cooking "light," keep a few tools of the trade on hand.

1. Nonstick cookware allows you to cut down on the amount of oil needed to sauté and brown foods.

2. Add moisture without adding fat by using broth, flavored vinegar, juice or wine in place of cream, butter and oil.

3. Make fat work harder. A dash of flavored oil or a sprinkle of a strong full-fat cheese like Parmesan, feta or blue cheese packs a lot of flavor into a recipe without loading on the fat. The key is to use a light touch.

Examples of LIGHT ways to prepare foods:

• Bake, broil, barbecue, microwave and grill.

• Substitute applesauce for 1/3 to 1/2 of the oil, butter or margarine in baked goods.

• Substitute fat-free or reduced-fat sour cream or cream cheese for regular versions.

LESS: Eat high-fat favorites less often and in smaller amounts

Don't toss out your favorite family recipes because they scream "too high in fat." You have options: make your favorites as usual and have smaller portions or serve them less often, or modify your favorite family recipes by reducing the fat and calories they contain.

Examples of LESS:

- Sprinkle cakes with powdered sugar rather than slathering them with frosting.

- Split a dessert with a friend.

- Decide to make your famous triple-layer chocolate cake only at holidays.

Making Food Lean, Light or Less

Pull out a few days of a current or old FOOD & ACTIVITY JOURNAL. Take five minutes to review this record and write down three ways that you could make your food choices LEAN, LIGHT and/or LESS.

1.

2.

3.

Recipe Makeovers

 Don't fall into the trap of trying to change too much at once. If you make drastic changes, you're more likely to revert back to your old habits. Progress slowly as you experiment with reducing the fat in your favorite recipes. Stop before you reach the point where you, or your family, won't eat it. You'll need to experiment to find a balance between good taste and what's good for you.

R.E.R.: A Formula for Recipe Makeovers
(Reduce, Eliminate, Replace)

Trim fat and calories from recipes by making adjustments in the ingredients and preparation methods you use.

Reduce high-fat/calorie ingredients

High fat ingredients: nuts, cheese, meat, oil, margarine, butter, cream, mayonnaise, sour cream, cream cheese, most cuts of red meat, dark meat of poultry.

Examples:
- In lasagna, reduce meat and high-fat cheeses to one-half the amount called for in the recipe.
- In stew, reduce meat to two ounces per serving.

Eliminate high-fat/calorie ingredients

Examples:
- In lasagna, eliminate meat and make it cheese lasagna.
- In stew, eliminate oil for browning meat and use a vegetable oil spray.

Replace high-fat/calorie ingredients with lower fat/calorie ingredients

Refer to the FIND A SUBSTITUTE! chart (page 176) for specific suggestions.

Examples:
- In lasagna, replace higher-fat cheeses with ones that are lower in fat; replace meat with spinach for vegetarian lasagna.
- In stew, replace part of the meat with more vegetables.

The following page shows an example of using the R.E.R. formula for trimming calories and fat from a Chicken Divan recipe.

Chicken Divan

Original Recipe

3 chicken breasts, halved and boned

1/3 cup butter

1 pound fresh asparagus spears

1 10-ounce can cream of chicken soup

2/3 cup mayonnaise

1/3 cup evaporated whole milk

2/3 cup grated cheddar cheese

1 tsp. lemon juice

1/2 tsp. curry powder

1/2 cup bread crumbs

1 Tbsp. butter

Brown chicken breasts in butter. Steam asparagus until crisp and tender. Arrange asparagus in baking dish; top with chicken.

Combine cream of chicken soup, mayonnaise, milk, cheese, lemon juice and curry. Pour over chicken. Sprinkle with bread crumbs. Dot with butter.

Bake at 350 degrees 40-45 minutes.
Yield: 6 servings

**Per serving: 625 calories
             48 grams of fat**

Converted Low-Fat Recipe

3 chicken breasts, halved, skinned and boned

1 pound fresh asparagus spears

1 10-ounce can reduced-fat cream of chicken soup

1/3 cup nonfat plain yogurt

1/3 cup skim evaporated milk

1/3 cup grated part-skim cheddar cheese

1 tsp. lemon juice

1/2 tsp. curry powder

1/2 cup bread crumbs

Brown chicken breasts lightly in a non-stick skillet or use non-stick spray in pan. Steam asparagus until crisp and tender. Arrange asparagus in baking dish; top with chicken.

Combine cream of chicken soup, mayonnaise, yogurt, milk, cheese, lemon juice and curry. Pour over chicken. Sprinkle with bread crumbs.

Bake at 350 degrees 40-45 minutes.
Yield: 6 servings

**Per serving: 285 calories
             10 grams of fat**

Effects of Low-Fat Modification

Instead of:	Change to:	Approximate grams of fat saved per serving
Chicken with skin	Chicken without skin	4
Browned in butter	Non-stick skillet	10
Regular cream of chicken soup	Reduced-fat cream of chicken soup	3
2/3 cup mayonnaise	1/3 cup reduced-calorie mayonnaise; 1/3 cup nonfat plain yogurt	16
1/3 cup evaporated whole milk	1/3 cup evaporated skim milk	1
2/3 cup cheddar cheese	1/3 cup part-skim cheddar cheese	2
Dot with butter (1 Tbsp.)	No butter	2
	TOTAL:	**38**

Source: Guidelines for Heart-Healthy Eating, Providence Health System, 1997.

Find a Substitute!

TRADITIONAL INGREDIENT	LOWER-FAT INGREDIENT
Whole Milk	Nonfat or lower-fat milk (1% or 2%), evaporated skim milk.
Cream	Nonfat or lower-fat milk (1% or 2%), nonfat plain yogurt or sour cream. Blended reduced-fat cottage cheese or evaporated skim milk. (Can be thickened with corn starch or vegetable puree.)
Cheese	Part skim or fat-free ricotta cheese or cottage cheese, lower-fat cheese (6 grams of fat or less per ounce), smaller amounts of strong-flavored cheeses such as Parmesan, Romano or extra-sharp cheddar. (*Tip:* grated cheese goes farther.)
Sour Cream	Nonfat or light sour cream, plain nonfat yogurt, buttermilk, reduced-fat cottage cheese blended with milk, yogurt cheese (plain yogurt strained through cheesecloth overnight).
Cream Cheese	Fat-free or light cream cheese, Neufchatel.
Whole Eggs	Egg whites, egg substitutes. (*Tip:* substitute two egg whites for one whole egg.)
Butter, margarine	For sautéing: nonstick vegetable oil sprays or a light brush of oil.
	For sauces & bases: stock or broth, water, wine, vegetable and fruit juices, liquid oils (no more than one teaspoon per serving).
Oil	Vegetable stock or nonstick vegetable oil spray.
Salad dressing	Replace two parts oil with chicken stock, fruit juice or flavored vinegar (balsamic, rice vinegar) or use nonfat yogurt as a base.
Mayonnaise	Light or fat-free mayonnaise, blended light or fat-free cream cheese.

Source: Adapted from The American Dietetic Association, 1994.

Meal Ideas: Quick, Easy and Tasty

Too tired to cook? Short on time? Prepare tasty and wholesome meals in minutes using convenience products.

Baked Potato with Toppings

Cook potatoes in the microwave. Allow four minutes for one medium potato and add two minutes for each additional potato.

Toppings: low-fat cheese and salsa, low-fat chili or baked beans, low-fat cottage cheese

Veggie Burgers

Look for this tasty sandwich option in the frozen food section of most grocery stores and health food stores. Try it on a toasted bun with "the works."

Soups and Low-fat Top Ramen

Start with canned or dehydrated varieties. Good soup bets: bean, rice, vegetable, lentil and couscous. To reduce sodium and boost the nutritional content, add leftover rice or pasta; canned, rinsed beans; or frozen vegetables.

Hot Dogs & Beans

Many brands of franks exist, even some vegetarian varieties (soy dogs). Read the label and look for brands with two grams of fat or less per frank. Serve with your favorite baked beans.

Macaroni & Cheese (and similar pasta products)

Prepare without the margarine; just add an extra dash of milk. Seek out brands that don't have a long list of artificial colors and flavorings.

Bean Burrito

Spread nonfat refried beans on a tortilla and microwave. Or place beans in the middle of the tortilla, fold the tortilla, and bake at 400 degrees for 10 minutes.

Toppings: low-fat cheese, salsa, light sour cream, lettuce and tomato

Pasta with Tomato Sauce

Cook pasta, heat sauce and eat. For flavor and a burst of nutrition, add veggies to the sauce such as onions, green or red pepper, broccoli or mushrooms.

Quick cooking pasta: angel hair pasta, fresh pasta

Quickie Side Dishes:

Fresh fruit with yogurt	Cucumbers with rice vinegar
Canned/frozen veggies	Baby carrots
Prewashed spinach/lettuce	Preshredded cabbage

Note: Refer to the Selected Resources section in the Appendix for cookbooks, cooking magazines and videos.

Navigating Roadblocks to Fitness

 You'll encounter plenty of obstacles on the road to better fitness. Here's a list of simple solutions to some common problems.

I don't have time.

Solution: Make your workout a priority. Examine obligations that eat up your time and energy. What's important? What can you give up, delegate or eliminate to make more room in your schedule? Also, the more active you are, the more energy you'll have to accomplish your daily tasks.

I'm too tired at the end of the day.

Solution: Exercise in the morning or try a noontime workout. Right after work may be a good time, too. If you choose this option, try to exercise before heading home. That way, family, pets, phones or the couch won't distract you from your plan.

I get injured.

Solution: Listen to your body. Be sure to start out gradually and go at a pace that feels right for you. When you finish, cool down with a few minutes of gentle stretching. Wear appropriate athletic shoes with good support. If you continue to have problems, see a sports medicine physician for advice.

The weather is bad.

Solution: If you tend to exercise outdoors, you need to have a "plan B" for nasty weather. Plan B can be attending a club, fitness class or indoor pool, or switching to a sport or activity more appropriate for the weather (for example, hiking with snowshoes instead of jogging). A piece of home exercise equipment or a fitness video can also do the trick.

I travel a lot.

Solution: Choose hotels that have a fitness center. Or pack your walking shoes and check with the front desk for recommendations on safe walking routes.

I get discouraged.

Solution: Check your expectations. Do you expect to look like Arnold after a few weight-lifting sessions? It takes time to see results. In the interim, reward yourself for small goals you achieve. (Reward ideas: fitness magazine, exercise clothing, CD, book, etc.) Chart your exercise, take credit for your efforts and be proud of your progress.

My S.M.A.R.T. Plans for this Week

Stop and take a few minutes to set up S.M.A.R.T. fitness and food plans for yourself this week. They may be the same or different than last week's plans.

S.M.A.R.T. FITNESS PLAN	S.M.A.R.T. FOOD PLAN
Specific What activity(s) will I do? Time of day? (a.m. or p.m.) **Measurable** How many days will I exercise? Which days will I exercise? How many minutes will I do it for? **Achievable** Is this plan realistic? Reasonable? **Relevant** Is this an activity I enjoy? Can I make it a priority this week? **Trackable** Where will I record my activity?	**Specific** What will I work on? **Measurable** How many days will I do it for? Which days will I target? (weekdays, weekends) **Achievable** Is this plan realistic? Reasonable? **Relevant** Will changing this eating habit make a difference in my health? **Trackable** How will I monitor this behavior?

Skill Practice: Week Seven

 Continue on the path to a healthier lifestyle by targeting some time to all four key areas (food, fitness, emotional support and planning) this week.

1. **Keep records** —Keep track of your eating habits using one of the following methods. Check one option or create your own tracking system.

   ☐ Record food only.

   ☐ Record food and hunger/fullness cues.

   ☐ Use the Food Pyramid for a nutrition check. (See Appendix.)

   ☐ Record food and calories.

   ☐ Record food and fat grams.

   ☐ Record your feelings before each meal or snack.

   ☐ My own tracking system

        (specify): _____

2. **Change distorted self-talk into balanced self-talk** — Challenge any negative self-talk you encounter this week with balanced self-talk. Record your negative thoughts and positive statements on the COUNTERING NEGATIVE SELF-TALK WORKSHEET provided on page 168.

3. **Try a new cooking or eating strategy** — Cook and eat "smarter" this week by using one new LEAN, LIGHT or LESS technique. Write down one or two ideas you plan to try this week:

4. **S.M.A.R.T. plans** — Follow the fitness and food plans you made for yourself this week.

Reminder: Don't forget to record your fitness activities in your FOOD & ACTIVITY JOURNAL.

FOOD & ACTIVITY JOURNAL

Date:_____

Day: M   Tu   W   Th   F   Sat   Sun

Fitness Activity:

TIME	FEELINGS CHECK	H/F SCALE*	FOOD & DRINK	AMOUNT	CALORIES	FAT (grams)	H/F SCALE*
					Total:	Total:	

*Rate your hunger/fullness on a scale from 0–10: 0 = Empty, 5 = Just Right, 10 = Stuffed

FOOD & ACTIVITY JOURNAL

Date:_____

Day: M   Tu   W   Th   F   Sat   Sun

Fitness Activity:

TIME	FEELINGS CHECK	H/F SCALE*	FOOD & DRINK	AMOUNT	CALORIES	FAT (grams)	H/F SCALE*
					Total:	Total:	

*Rate your hunger/fullness on a scale from 0–10: 0 = Empty, 5 = Just Right, 10 = Stuffed

FOOD & ACTIVITY JOURNAL

Date:_____

Day: M   Tu   W   Th   F   Sat   Sun

Fitness Activity:	

TIME	FEELINGS CHECK	H/F SCALE*	FOOD & DRINK	AMOUNT	CALORIES	FAT (grams)	H/F SCALE*
					Total:	Total:	

*Rate your hunger/fullness on a scale from 0–10: 0 = Empty, 5 = Just Right, 10 = Stuffed

FOOD & ACTIVITY JOURNAL

Date:_____

Day: M   Tu   W   Th   F   Sat   Sun

Fitness Activity:

TIME	FEELINGS CHECK	H/F SCALE*	FOOD & DRINK	AMOUNT	CALORIES	FAT (grams)	H/F SCALE*
					Total:	Total:	

*Rate your hunger/fullness on a scale from 0–10: 0 = Empty, 5 = Just Right, 10 = Stuffed

FOOD & ACTIVITY JOURNAL

Date:_____

Day: M Tu W Th F Sat Sun

Fitness Activity:

TIME	FEELINGS CHECK	H/F SCALE*	FOOD & DRINK	AMOUNT	CALORIES	FAT (grams)	H/F SCALE*
					Total:	Total:	

*Rate your hunger/fullness on a scale from 0–10: 0 = Empty, 5 = Just Right, 10 = Stuffed

FOOD & ACTIVITY JOURNAL

Date:_____

Day: M   Tu   W   Th   F   Sat   Sun

Fitness Activity:

TIME	FEELINGS CHECK	H/F SCALE*	FOOD & DRINK	AMOUNT	CALORIES	FAT (grams)	H/F SCALE*
					Total:	Total:	

*Rate your hunger/fullness on a scale from 0–10: 0 = Empty, 5 = Just Right, 10 = Stuffed

FOOD & ACTIVITY JOURNAL

Date:_____

Day: M   Tu   W   Th   F   Sat   Sun

Fitness Activity:	

TIME	FEELINGS CHECK	H/F SCALE*	FOOD & DRINK	AMOUNT	CALORIES	FAT (grams)	H/F SCALE*
					Total:	Total:	

*Rate your hunger/fullness on a scale from 0–10: 0 = Empty, 5 = Just Right, 10 = Stuffed

Stay Young in Mind and Body

Only you can manage your weight and take control of your health. Do you meet this responsibility head on? How many times have you lost weight for your spouse, parents or an upcoming reunion or wedding? What happened after you lost the weight? Losing weight to please others or for a special event usually doesn't produce the long-term results most people are looking for. Why not? Losing weight for someone or something else provides a temporary boost at best.

Look at people who have lost weight and kept it off. They find their efforts to be most effective once they decide to do it for themselves. The best way to motivate yourself to change is to find a reason from within. Work on accepting what you can't change. Move on and take charge of the things you can change, like your overall body size, your fitness level and your health.

This Week You Will:

- Reflect over the previous week, noting insights and accomplishments.
- Learn how to make smart food choices when dining out.
- Identify ways to enhance your feelings about your body (body acceptance).
- Discover ten mini-moves that will help you stay active.
- Design a personal S.M.A.R.T. plan for food and fitness.

Reflections

 ## Reflect on your FOOD & ACTIVITY JOURNAL

Which aspect(s) of your food intake/eating habits did you track? What did you learn from this activity?

Reflect on changing negative self-talk into balanced self-talk

What did you learn from writing down your negative thoughts and devising positive counter statements on the COUNTERING NEGATIVE SELF-TALK WORKSHEET?

Reflect on using LEAN, LIGHT and LESS techniques to make healthier food choices

Which technique(s) worked for you and why? Which didn't work and why?

Reflect on your S.M.A.R.T. plans

How did these plans work for you? Do you plan to use them again, throw them out or fine-tune them?

Other observations from last week

What worked well for you? What didn't work?

Check, Please!

Eating out, a great American pastime, provides a welcome break from the hustle and bustle of our daily lives. It's a time to enjoy the company of family and friends, and an opportunity to experience ethnic foods and new flavor combinations.

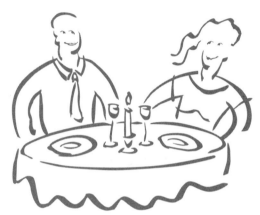

Whether you splurge or budget your calories when you dine at a restaurant depends on the occasion and how often you dine out. An occasional night of indulging won't undo all the healthy choices you make day to day. But the average American eats 20 percent of his or her meals away from home. If you dine out several times a week, you need to be making smart choices.

Eating Healthy Away from Home

1. Plan Ahead

Select a restaurant that offers a variety of healthy options: Chinese, Japanese, Indian, seafood or vegetarian restaurants.

Never arrive ravenously hungry — it leads to overeating. When you slip down to a "0" or "1" on the HUNGER/FULLNESS SCALE, it can be hard to resist diving into the basket of bread or chips.

If you plan to indulge, take measures for damage control. Eat lighter (but don't skip meals) during the day and pick up the pace of your exercise for a few days either before or after your night on the town.

2. Have it Your Way

A good restaurant wants satisfied customers. Don't be afraid to ask questions about how foods are prepared and the ingredients they contain. Enlist the help of the waitress or waiter to make sure you get what you want.

- Request that foods be prepared with less fat.

    May I please have dry toast with jam or honey on the side?

    Can the shrimp be sautéed in wine instead of fried?

    May I please have the salad dressing (or butter, gravy, sauce) served on the side?

- Substitute foods that have less fat and fewer calories.

  May I have a baked potato instead of fries?

  May I have the salad with salad dressing "on the side" in place of coleslaw?

- Consider using nonfat condiments such as freshly squeezed lemon, salsa or flavored vinegar in lieu of butter, margarine and sour cream.

3. Practice Portion Control

- To control portions, order a la carte or request a "half order" or a child's portion.

- Be creative — order soup or an appetizer(s) instead of an entree. For example, a bowl of minestrone soup or a shrimp cocktail, salad and fresh bread may really hit the spot.

- Restaurant portions can be too large to eat at one sitting. Consider taking half or part of your meal home. Get in the habit of requesting a doggie bag.

- Split an entree with a friend and order a salad. Or share the chocolate raspberry cheesecake that you've been craving — it provides only half the fat and calories when you split it with someone.

4. Pay Attention to Your Body

Watch the pace at which you eat. Slow down and enjoy the taste, texture and aroma of your food. If you find yourself scanning the dessert menu while others savor their entrees, slow down and match the pace of a slower eater at the table.

Pay special attention to hunger and fullness cues when dining out. No one enjoys feeling stuffed. It's uncomfortable. Strive to leave the restaurant feeling satisfied but without having to unbutton your pants or loosen your belt a couple of notches.

Low-fat Menu Lingo

Steamed	Grilled	Baked
Garden fresh	Poached	Broiled
Flame cooked	Stir-fried	Roasted

High-fat Menu Lingo

Crispy	Tempura	Cheese sauce
Au gratin	Breaded	Fried, batter fried, pan fried
Flaky	Hollandaise	Creamy

Smart Food Guide To Restaurants

MEXICAN

Decide what you want to spend your calories on — the chips, marguerites or the dinner? You'll leave the restaurant feeling stuffed and uncomfortable, as well as way over your calorie-fat budget, if you feast on all of them. Watch out for guacamole, sour cream and shredded cheese; these foods come loaded with fat. Ask for flour or corn tortillas in place of greasy fried shells.

Smart choices:
- Chicken or bean tostadas
- Arroz con pollo (chicken with rice)
- Arroz con camaron (shrimp with rice)
- Fajitas
- Kebabs
- Chicken or bean burritos
- Black beans
- Tacos
- Low-fat sauces: salsa, pico de gallo

CHINESE AND ASIAN

Choose broiled, steamed or lightly stir-fried dishes. Watch out for the fat in fried rice and in the egg foo yung, sweet 'n' sour, crispy and deep-fried dishes.

Smart choices:
- Stir-fried meat, poultry or seafood mixed with vegetables
- Chow mein
- Teriyaki
- Steamed rice
- Chop suey
- Broth soups

DELI FOOD

Watch out for mayonnaise, oil and special sauces. Choose whole-grain bagels, rolls and bread over croissants for sandwiches. Beware of mayonnaise and oil in pasta and potato salads.

Smart choices:
- Sandwich of lean meats, topped with vegetables
- Green or fruit salads
- Soups: broth-based, lentil, bean

ITALIAN

Beware of the cheese, cream sauces (e.g., Alfredo) and the oversized portions!

Smart choices:

- Low-fat sauces: marsala (wine) and marinara (tomatoes, onions, garlic)
- Pasta with red clam, mussel sauce or marinara sauce
- Pasta primavera
- Minestrone soup
- Pizza or calzone with vegetable or shrimp toppings (request less cheese)
- Chicken or seafood cacciatore
- Cioppino (seafood soup)
- Veal with wine sauce
- Spinach and ricotta cheese ravioli or manicotti topped with tomato sauce

GREEK

Avoid deep-fried falafel. Ask for dishes to be served without olive oil, which is often used as a topping.

Smart choices:

- Meat and vegetable shish kebab
- Couscous
- Pilafs
- Tabbouleh

FRENCH

Enjoy fresh French bread — it tastes great without butter. Ask for sauces to be served on the side. Beware of high-fat fondues, quiches and cream sauces.

Smart choices:

- Bouillabaisse
- Coq au vin (chicken in wine sauce)
- Poached salmon
- Poulet aux fines herbes (roast chicken with herbs)
- Steamed mussels or clams

AIRLINE TRAVEL

Most airlines offer alternative meals to health-conscious passengers at no extra cost. Simply request your special meal when you reserve your seat.

Eating on the Run

Do you often find yourself hungry, but short on time? You may be running errands or enjoying vacation sights, for example, and simply want to refuel quickly. Try to plan ahead by bringing snacks in the car (bagels, string cheese, apples), but don't worry if you find yourself limited to grocery stores or fast food restaurants for a quick bite — plenty of healthy options exist for you to choose from.

GROCERY/CONVENIENCE STORES

Many grocery stores offer sandwiches from the deli, a salad bar in the produce section and even a take-out Chinese food area.

Smart choices:

- Yogurt
- Fresh fruit (apples, oranges, bananas, grapes)
- Bagels with light cream cheese
- Reduced-fat crackers and low-fat cheese
- Rice bowl with stir-fry (if Chinese take-out is available)
- Fruit juice
- Deli-style sandwiches
- Salad/soup bar

FAST FOOD RESTAURANTS

Watch out for "jumbo," "super-sized," "double" or "triple" foods and beverages; they just mean more calories. Ask for a copy of the nutrition information for your favorite foods. Most fast food restaurants will have it posted, but if they don't, call and obtain it from their headquarters.

Smart choices:

- Plain burger with catsup, mustard, relish, vegetables (to really cut the fat: select the smallest burger, skip the cheese, and hold the mayo or special sauce)
- Grilled chicken sandwich (hold the mayo; try barbecue sauce instead)
- Low-fat deli sandwiches (turkey, lean roast beef, lean ham), add veggies and mustard but hold the mayo and the oil
- Pizza with shrimp, plain cheese or vegetables (ask for half the amount of cheese)
- Baked potato with chili or cottage cheese (watch cheesy toppings)
- Chili
- Low-fat milk or fruit juice

Grabbing Fast Food from the Low-Fat Lane

Take five minutes and write down three "on the run" meals that would work for you. Make sure the meals include foods you like and have enough calories to be satisfying.

1.

2.

3.

Body Acceptance Begins at Home

 In today's world, judgments about weight are pervasive. In fact, size discrimination or prejudice against large-sized people is commonly referred to as *weightism*. Keep your eye out for weightism. Sometimes it's obvious, as in name-calling and social ridicule. But weightism can manifest itself more subtly with job discrimination or subpar medical care.

We all need to be sensitive to the devastating effects of weightism. Bodies come in a variety of shapes and sizes. We need to respect these differences, just as we do with age, gender, skin color and ethnic backgrounds.

How to Recover Your Body Acceptance

You were born feeling comfortable with your body. You accepted your chubby legs and double chin without judgment. Over the years, unrealistic pressure from society combined with your own personal experiences may have forced you to become uncomfortable with your body. When this happens, the self-acceptance you knew as a child turns to self-rejection as an adult.

Your self-esteem and how you view your body (your body image) are strongly linked. Sometimes you may be hard on yourself in the hopes that it will motivate you to make changes. Your inner critical voice may sound like this: *I'm so fat; look at that stomach!* But this strategy will only backfire. How can you feel motivated to take good care of your body if you don't like it or are critical of it? Learning to accept and respect your body forms the foundation you need in order to make positive changes in your behaviors.

Instrumental vs. Ornamental

Not a day goes by that we don't receive messages about how our bodies should look — from TV, magazines, movies, newspapers, clothing sizes, family members and even complete strangers. It's easy to see how we've come to view our bodies as ornaments rather than instruments. We think our looks (external) matter more than what is on the inside (internal). We even take it a step further and project specific attributes to certain physical features. We assume that all slender, pretty women are happy, for example, and that tall men with athletic builds must be successful. We fantasize about thinner thighs, firmer bodies and flatter tummies. How did we get to this place?

Mirror, Mirror on the Wall

Here's what can happen if you emotionally react to the perfect standards the media and today's society try to sell us on:

- You reject your body. This wounds your self-esteem.
- You never feel good enough.
- You stop listening to your body, start ignoring internal messages.
- You focus on the external rather than the internal (how you feel).
- You let someone else define who you are or who you should be.

How can you focus on seeing and experiencing your body as an instrument rather than an ornament? It's simple — stop and think about it. Your body serves you in many ways. You may not appreciate the appearance of your legs, but you can be grateful for the ability to walk and get to where you need to go. Let's face it, your body wouldn't function the same without legs.

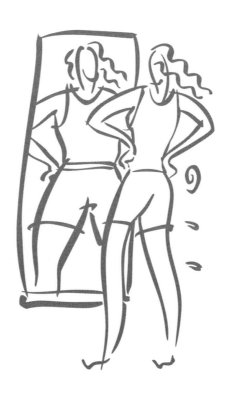

Take five minutes right now and explore some of the other ways that your body serves you. First, identify those body parts that you have negative thoughts about. Next, counter your negative feelings with positive statements about the functions of that body part, or how it serves you.

BODY PART	INSTRUMENTAL: POSITIVE FUNCTION(S)
Example: Nose	I breathe through my nose. I can smell the delicious aromas of ethnic foods and the scent of spring flowers.

Next time you find yourself being critical of these body parts, focus on the positive aspects you just identified. It may feel awkward at first as you relearn to appreciate and respect your body, but it gets easier with practice.

Promoting Body Acceptance

Want to feel better about your body? Focus on the following concepts.

1. Confront weightism.

Challenge any negative thoughts you have about your own weight, but at the same time, don't be too hard on yourself when you notice this negativity. Weightism permeates our society, so naturally it's going to rub off on you and others in your life. Increasing your awareness can help you question and distance yourself from harmful messages.

Seek out health care providers who hold informed and sensitive attitudes about weight issues. This means finding providers who respect you and listen to your needs and concerns. Interactions shouldn't leave you feeling ashamed, defensive or misunderstood.

Notice the attitudes toward weight that the people around you express, in particular your family and friends. If you feel comfortable, share your feelings about weightism.

2. Spend time with people who respect and support you.

This means people who:

- Care more about how you feel than about how you look.
- Respect that you control your own weight and food choices.
- Don't react to changes in your weight by becoming either more distant or more friendly.
- Do not make rude or intrusive comments about your choices regarding weight, eating, exercise and/or personal appearance.

Seek out positive "large-size" role models (people you know, famous people and size-friendly magazines, for example). Focus on those who participate in life, feel good about themselves, enjoy their bodies, and make meaningful contributions to the world.

3. Notice cultural influences on weight and size.

Our culture's narrow and unrealistic definition of beauty and health doesn't serve any useful purpose. Broaden your horizons by looking at pictures of the human body in art, in different cultures and in different historical eras.

Notice when people make assumptions about another person's inner qualities based on their size and appearance. Weight has nothing to do with a person's moral character or basic worth. Wonderful (and not-so-wonderful) people come in all shapes and sizes.

4. Honor your body where it is now.

Allow yourself to accept compliments. When you do, you acknowledge your positive traits and characteristics. Practice giving compliments to others. By doing so, you acknowledge your opinion as being important and worthwhile to share with others.

Focus on feeling good in the body you have now. This means you should treat your body with the same level of care and generosity that you would if you were slender. Carry yourself in a way that conveys energy, confidence and pride in who you are. Do things that help you enjoy your body in sensory ways (e.g., massage, soak in a hot tub, cozy fabrics for clothing or bedding, fragrant candles, long relaxing shower or bath).

Whenever you feel bad about yourself or your weight, stop and check your self-talk. Replace any harsh or helpless-sounding phrases with something kinder and more encouraging.

Improving Body Acceptance

> **You deserve to be treated with respect and care, by yourself and by others. Take a few minutes and list one way in which you will work to improve your body acceptance this week. Refer to the preceding section for ideas.**

Ten Mini-Moves That Don't Require Tennis Shoes

 Every move you make counts toward burning fat and calories — even the small stuff! Here's a list of suggestions that can help you keep moving in between your planned fitness activities.

1. Walk up instead of driving up to your bank, dry cleaner or favorite coffee haunt.

2. Use the stairs instead of the elevator. Too many floors to tackle? Hit the stairs for several flights and hitch a ride on the elevator for the remaining floors.

3. Retire the remote control. Get up to switch channels on the TV or to turn down the volume on your stereo.

4. Walk to the store, school or park instead of hopping in your car.

5. Don't delegate your activity. You be the one to get the mail, put the garbage out or walk the dog.

6. Park your car farther away from your destination any chance you get (shopping trips, dental and doctor appointments, movies, etc.).

7. If you take the bus, get off a few stops early and walk the rest of the way.

8. Shopping at the mall? Walk a loop around the perimeter before going into any stores.

9. If you arrive early to an appointment, take advantage of the extra time and go for a walk. *Tip:* Always carry a pair of walking shoes in your trunk.

10. Dig in the yard. Gardening and yard work offer many opportunities for you to move — aside from being fit, you'll have a beautiful yard.

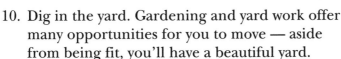

My S.M.A.R.T. Plans for this Week

Stop and take a few minutes to set up S.M.A.R.T. fitness and food plans for yourself this week. They may be the same or different than last week's plans.

S.M.A.R.T. FITNESS PLAN
Specific What activity(s) will I do?
Time of day? (a.m. or p.m.)
Measurable How many days will I exercise?
Which days will I exercise?
How many minutes will I do it for?
Achievable Is this plan realistic? Reasonable?
Relevant Is this an activity I enjoy?
Can I make it a priority this week?
Trackable Where will I record my activity?

S.M.A.R.T. FOOD PLAN
Specific What will I work on?
Measurable How many days will I do it for?
Which days will I target? (weekdays, weekends)
Achievable Is this plan realistic? Reasonable?
Relevant Will changing this eating habit make a difference in my health?
Trackable How will I monitor this behavior?

Skill Practice: Week Eight

 Life throws challenges at us every day, like eating healthy meals away from home or defending ourselves against weightism (weight discrimination). Prepare yourself for these situations by developing the necessary skills now.

1. **Keep records** —Keep track of your eating habits using one of the following methods. Check one option or create your own tracking system.

   ☐ Record food only.

   ☐ Record food and hunger/fullness cues.

   ☐ Use the Food Pyramid for a nutrition check. (See Appendix.)

   ☐ Record food and calories.

   ☐ Record food and fat grams.

   ☐ Record your feelings before each meal or snack.

   ☐ My own tracking system

   (specify): _____

2. **Practice making smart food choices in a restaurant** — Plan to eat away from home sometime within the next week or two. Practice using one or two tips introduced in the "Check, Please!" (dining out) section of this chapter or try a new "on the run" meal (see page 197).

3. **Enhance your feelings about your body** — Follow through with the activity you selected for improving your body acceptance (see page 202).

4. **S.M.A.R.T. plans** — Follow the fitness and food plans you made for yourself this week.

> *Reminder:* Don't forget to record your fitness activities in your FOOD & ACTIVITY JOURNAL.

FOOD & ACTIVITY JOURNAL

Date:_____

Day: M   Tu   W   Th   F   Sat   Sun

Fitness Activity:

TIME	FEELINGS CHECK	H/F SCALE*	FOOD & DRINK	AMOUNT	CALORIES	FAT (grams)	H/F SCALE*
					Total:	Total:	

*Rate your hunger/fullness on a scale from 0–10: 0 = Empty, 5 = Just Right, 10 = Stuffed

FOOD & ACTIVITY JOURNAL

Date:_____

Day: M   Tu   W   Th   F   Sat   Sun

Fitness Activity:

TIME	FEELINGS CHECK	H/F SCALE*	FOOD & DRINK	AMOUNT	CALORIES	FAT (grams)	H/F SCALE*
					Total:	Total:	

*Rate your hunger/fullness on a scale from 0–10: 0 = Empty, 5 = Just Right, 10 = Stuffed

FOOD & ACTIVITY JOURNAL

Date:_____

Day: M Tu W Th F Sat Sun

Fitness Activity:

TIME	FEELINGS CHECK	H/F SCALE*	FOOD & DRINK	AMOUNT	CALORIES	FAT (grams)	H/F SCALE*
					Total:	Total:	

*Rate your hunger/fullness on a scale from 0–10: 0 = Empty, 5 = Just Right, 10 = Stuffed

FOOD & ACTIVITY JOURNAL

Date:_____

Day: M   Tu   W   Th   F   Sat   Sun

Fitness Activity:	

TIME	FEELINGS CHECK	H/F SCALE*	FOOD & DRINK	AMOUNT	CALORIES	FAT (grams)	H/F SCALE*
					Total:	Total:	

*Rate your hunger/fullness on a scale from 0–10: 0 = Empty, 5 = Just Right, 10 = Stuffed

FOOD & ACTIVITY JOURNAL

Date:_____

Day: M   Tu   W   Th   F   Sat   Sun

Fitness Activity:

TIME	FEELINGS CHECK	H/F SCALE*	FOOD & DRINK	AMOUNT	CALORIES	FAT (grams)	H/F SCALE*
					Total:	Total:	

*Rate your hunger/fullness on a scale from 0–10: 0 = Empty, 5 = Just Right, 10 = Stuffed

FOOD & ACTIVITY JOURNAL

Date:_____

Day: M   Tu   W   Th   F   Sat   Sun

Fitness Activity:	

TIME	FEELINGS CHECK	H/F SCALE*	FOOD & DRINK	AMOUNT	CALORIES	FAT (grams)	H/F SCALE*
					Total:	Total:	

*Rate your hunger/fullness on a scale from 0–10: 0 = Empty, 5 = Just Right, 10 = Stuffed

FOOD & ACTIVITY JOURNAL

Date:_____

Day:　M　Tu　W　Th　F　Sat　Sun

Fitness Activity:	

TIME	FEELINGS CHECK	H/F SCALE*	FOOD & DRINK	AMOUNT	CALORIES	FAT (grams)	H/F SCALE*
					Total:	Total:	

*Rate your hunger/fullness on a scale from 0–10: 0 = Empty, 5 = Just Right, 10 = Stuffed

New Directions

There's no doubt about it. Losing weight and keeping it off requires hard work. Some people secretly believe they can return to their former eating habits once they reach their goal weight. But it doesn't work that way. Keeping the weight off permanently requires a lifelong commitment to a new way of living. It may sound overwhelming, but many people have done it and you can too. Continue to practice the new skills you have learned over the past several weeks. Take it one day at a time. Days turn into weeks, weeks lead to months, and months turn into years of healthy living.

> **This Week You Will:**
>
> - Reflect over the previous week, noting insights and accomplishments.
> - Recognize the importance of asserting yourself in eating situations.
> - Anticipate and plan for obstacles that arise in social eating situations.
> - Put a new spin on your fitness routine to prevent boredom or burnout.
> - Design a personal S.M.A.R.T. plan for food and fitness.

Reflections

 ### Reflect on your FOOD & ACTIVITY JOURNAL

Which aspect(s) of your food intake/eating habits did you track last week? What did you learn from this activity?

Reflect on making smarter food choices in restaurants

If you had an opportunity to eat out this past week, which techniques did you practice with regard to eating less or making lower-fat selections? Would you use them again?

Reflect on body acceptance

What did you do to enhance your body acceptance this past week? What observations did you make regarding weightism (weight discrimination)?

Reflect on your S.M.A.R.T. plans

How did these plans work for you? Do you plan to use them again, throw them out or fine-tune them?

Other observations from last week
What worked well for you? What didn't work?

Don't Be Afraid to Speak Up!

 In a typical year, based on eating three meals a day, you decide whether or not to eat more than one thousand times! The decision to eat is yours and yours alone. No one can coax you into eating unless you allow them to. Your job is to recognize and acknowledge that you have rights in social eating situations. You need to speak up to "food pushers" and address belittling remarks made by others or yourself. Take a look at the chart below to see how your behavior can influence the decisions you make about food and your health.

Around Your Health: Are You Passive, Assertive or Aggressive?

	PASSIVE	**ASSERTIVE**	**AGGRESSIVE**
What it Means	You allow others to treat you, and your thoughts and feelings, in whatever manner they want without a challenge.	You think and act in a manner that honors your legitimate personal rights.	You stand up for what you want regardless of the rights and feelings of others.
	You do what others want you to do regardless of your own desires.	You acknowledge and respect the rights of others.	You bully or humiliate others to get what you want.
	I'm not OK, you are.	I'm OK, you're OK.	I'm OK, you're not.
View of Rights	You view the rights of others as superior to your own. You're reluctant to assert your rights and privileges.	You're aware of your rights and privileges and recognize them as equal to the rights of others.	You view your rights as superior to the rights of others.
	You allow your rights to be violated by others or you ignore your own rights.	You take responsibility for your feelings and behaviors.	You often violate the rights of others.
Self-Expression	You don't express feelings and opinions directly, and you often repress your true feelings.	You express your feelings and opinions directly.	You express your feelings and opinions directly; you often manipulate others by blaming or intimidating them.
Food	You eat to please others.	You turn down food without explanation or guilt.	You turn down food with a demeaning remark.
Support	You hope or maybe hint at your need for support.	You request support.	You demand support.
Weight	You're reluctant to accept responsibility for your weight problem.	You accept responsibility for your weight problem.	You blame others for your weight problem.

Whether you behave in a passive, assertive or aggressive manner depends on the situation and the circumstances. You may be assertive, for example, when you discuss the vacation menu with your family. On the other hand, you may sit back passively when your mother-in-law makes plans for the next holiday celebration.

What impact do these behaviors have on your weight and health? Take a moment and think about it. If you tend to be passive in social situations that involve food, you simply eat whatever someone serves you, whether you want it or not. Emotional overeating often stems from these situations because you ignore your thoughts and feelings (a form of passive behavior). Instead of speaking up and expressing yourself, you tend to stuff your thoughts and feelings down with food. At the other end of the scale, if you act aggressively and demand that your family support you in your efforts to eat lower-fat foods, they may do so begrudgingly. As their resentment builds, you find the support you receive from family members sliding away.

To find a happy medium, you need to be assertive and stand up for yourself. This doesn't mean you have to be loud or offensive when you voice your opinion. You simply need to express your thoughts and feelings in a clear, direct and respectful manner. Take a look and see how assertive communication works in the following situation.

Example: Friend or relative says: *"Have some cake. I baked it just for you."*

Passive reaction: Afraid of hurting the person's feelings, you eat a piece.

Aggressive reaction: You retort, *"I can't eat this cake, I'm on a diet. Furthermore, you shouldn't be eating this cake either."*

Assertive reaction: You evaluate whether or not you want a piece of cake. If the answer is NO, you respond: *"No, thank you."* If you answer YES, you plan it into your day's food intake. You may decide to have a smaller piece, or to share a piece with a friend.

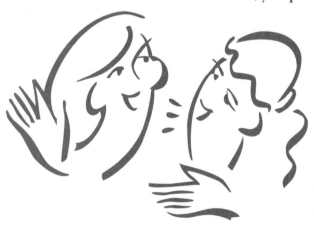

How to Be More Assertive

Many ways exist for you to be more assertive. Here are just a few to get you started:

- Believe that *you have a right* to good health and happiness. (The right to express your opinions and preferences, to say "no" and to make mistakes.)

- Let others know what you need. Tell them what's on your mind and how you feel.

- Make decisions that benefit your needs.

Use the following method to help you communicate your needs to others in a clear and assertive manner.

Speaking Up

Step one: Use feeling words to describe how the person's behavior affects you.
"I feel . . ."

Step two: Describe the outcome you desire.
"I want/need/prefer . . ."

Example:

1. *I feel* upset and angry when you bring me cookies.

2. *I need* your help in supporting my new eating habits. Please don't buy me any cookies unless I ask for them.

As with any other new skill you learn, it may take time and practice before you feel comfortable responding in an assertive manner. Others may even resist your new attitude. Be patient with these people and give them a chance to adapt to your new style of communication.

If you need help and support in this area, consider taking an assertiveness class or seek out a counselor who has experience in dealing with assertiveness issues.

Don't Let "Food Pushers" Push You Around

No matter how well you plan ahead or what strategies you arm yourself with, at some point, you will encounter the dreaded "food pusher." For whatever reason, these people thrive on getting you to eat what they want you to eat.

Keep these techniques in mind when you need to "push" back:

- Practice saying "no, thank you" gracefully. Sometimes, you have to repeat it over and over like a broken record. Stand firm on your decision.

- Use one-liners and avoid prolonged explanations. (It's your right not to have to justify yourself to others.)

    Examples:

    I'm full. I'm not hungry right now. Thanks, I've had enough. It was delicious but I'm stuffed. Maybe later. Thanks but no thanks.

When food represents love, the situation tends to be more complex. You need to be sensitive to the other person's feelings without giving away your right to good health. Be sure to acknowledge this person in a positive way. You can be loving and reassuring without having to stuff yourself.

Examples:

Grandma, I love your cooking, but I've had enough.

You're a fabulous cook. I enjoyed every bite, but I'm done.

How to Deal with Social Eating Pressures

Take five minutes and reflect back on the last time you found yourself in a social eating situation and felt pressured to eat. How could you handle this situation differently in the future?

Survival Tips for Special Occasions

Holidays, birthdays, weddings, graduations, parties and anniversaries all provide opportunities for you to celebrate as well as overindulge. But you can't stick your head in the sand and hide from these events. Celebrating with family and friends is part of the joy of living. You need to think ahead and plan for these festive occasions. The key to success with social eating — act by planning ahead, don't just react.

When it comes to parties and holiday celebrations, for example, you don't need a crystal ball to foresee the future. You've been there before. Maybe you're one of the people who typically gains seven to ten pounds every year between Thanksgiving and New Year's. You can learn from past celebrations, they give you insight into your eating behaviors. Take a moment and think about last year's holiday season. If you were able to maintain your weight, what strategies helped you do so? If not, what could you have done differently? How can you use this knowledge to your benefit during upcoming celebrations?

Always consider your options when celebrating. Of course, you can simply indulge and enjoy the occasion without feeling guilty. Or you can balance the calorie equation by eating less and being more physically active for several days before and/or after the event. Another option is to develop a solid game plan for yourself. Try some new strategies and see what works best for you. If they work, you gain some new skills. If they don't work, you can always head back to the drawing board for a new plan. Here's a list of tips to help you plan ahead for holidays and other celebrations.

Plan Ahead

If family celebrations mean sitting at a table that is loaded with high-fat foods, offer to bring a low-fat appetizer or a healthy green salad. Budgeting your calories throughout the day also helps. You don't want to skip meals to save calories for an evening event. You'll end up on the low end of the HUNGER/FULLNESS SCALE, which sets you up to overeat. Instead, watch your portions and cut down on higher-fat foods and condiments.

Strategies for Celebrations

Before:

- Never arrive hungry. You'll have to fight your hunger and tempting foods at the same time. Have a mini-meal (e.g., a piece of fruit, yogurt, some vegetables or a glass of nonfat milk) before you have to confront a potentially fattening situation.

- Arrive a little late. This way you won't stand around nibbling and drinking just to feel less awkward or shy. You'll also spend less time in contact with food.

- Bring a low-fat hors d'oeuvre plate that you and other health-conscious party-goers can splurge on.

During:

- Before you slip something into your mouth, ask yourself: "Am I really hungry?" If not, socialize instead. If yes, pay attention to what you eat and enjoy it.

- Eye everything on the buffet table before you get in line. Decide ahead of time what favorites or special foods will make it onto your plate.

- Pass up ordinary foods. You can have chips and dip, bread, cheese and nuts any day. Spend your calories on something really special.

- Don't nibble from serving bowls or plates. Instead, place food on a plate so you know how much you're eating.

- SLOW DOWN! Make foods and beverages last. Take small bites and put your utensil down in between. Sipping on water between mouthfuls will also help you slow down.

- If foods look or smell overly tempting, move to a room where foods or drinks won't be served.

- Have a predetermined cut-off time for eating. You may decide, for example, not to eat anything after 8:30 p.m.

- Keep your hands full with a napkin and a glass of water or a low-calorie drink. This will help you reduce the number of times you reach for food or alcoholic drinks.

Beverages: WATCH THE ALCOHOL!

- Save calories by cutting down on the number of drinks you have. This will also help you pass up some of the extras you typically consume once the alcohol takes effect and reduces your ability to make wise choices.

- Mixes can add a lot of extra calories. Check out the difference in calories between a highball made with a mix (190 calories) and a whiskey and water (120 calories).

- Ice extends the life of a drink without adding any calories.

- Alternate alcoholic drinks with nonalcoholic beverages. You'll save calories by reducing your alcohol intake. Enjoy water, club soda or mineral water with a twist, diet soda, vegetable juices or fruit juices.

- Dilute alcohol and your calorie intake by choosing a wine spritzer (wine and soda water).

After:
- Send tempting leftovers home with a guest or freeze the food immediately for later use.

- If you have overindulged, don't let feelings of guilt trap you into abandoning your efforts to maintain or manage your weight. Instead, cut down on (but don't skip) the next few meals and get moving.

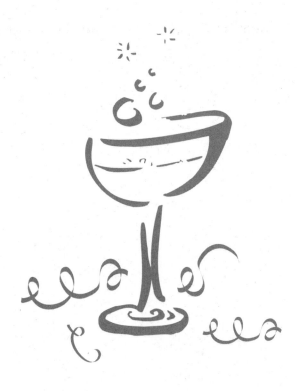

Planning for the Next Celebration

Drawing from your past experiences and the strategies listed on the previous pages, take five minutes to come up with a plan for how you might handle food at the next special celebration in your life (holiday, birthday, party, etc.).

My next celebration is:

My plan is to:

Potential barriers to this plan (what might get in my way?):

Possible solutions:

Put a New Spin on Your Fitness Program

It's easy to get bored doing the same old thing. A few bells and whistles may be all it takes to put a new spin on your fitness program.

- Challenge your limits. Sign up for a local fun walk or run, or spend a day on a guided walking tour or hiking trip. You'll have more fun if you take friends and family with you.

- Don't get stuck in a rut. Alternate your fitness routine. For example, walk briskly three days a week and cycle gently the other two.

- Try something new. Join the local pool or cycling club. Sign up for a new fitness class or give a new sport or activity a try. Ideas: yoga, martial arts, swing dance, mall walking, snowshoeing or cross-country skiing.

- Alter your route, or try your same route from the opposite direction. If you walk, jog or cycle, try a new route on weekends when you have more time. Vary the length and speed of your daily workouts.

- Jazz up your routine. Buy new athletic shoes, socks or clothing.

Try Something New

List one thing you will do this week to put a new spin on your fitness routine:

_____

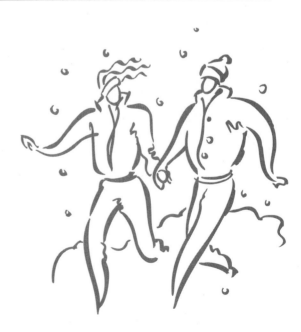

Water: The Overlooked Nutrient

Water! You can't live without it, but it's easily forgotten over the course of a busy day.

Water: It Does a Body Good

- Prevents dehydration.

- Takes the edge off hunger.

- Rids the body of toxins and waste products.

- Regulates the body's heating and cooling system.

- Plays a key role in digesting, absorbing and transporting nutrients.

When You Don't Get Enough

Dehydration results when your body runs low on fluid.

Signs of dehydration: headache, fatigue, dark urine (should be pale yellow), flushed skin, heat intolerance, light-headedness, dry mouth and eyes.

How Much Water Do You Need?

Drinking 8 to 12 cups per day is recommended. Be sure to count only noncaffeinated, nonalcoholic beverages. You require more water in warm weather, at higher altitudes and whenever you exercise.

A Toast to Your Health! Tips for Drinking More Water

- Get in the habit of carrying a water bottle with you. Put it where you can see it as a reminder to drink.

- Drink a glass with every meal.

- Drink before, during and after exercise.

- If water from your tap leaves a bad taste in your mouth, try a filter to improve the flavor.

My S.M.A.R.T. Plans for this Week

Stop and take a few minutes to set up S.M.A.R.T. fitness and food plans for yourself this week. They may be the same or different than last week's plans.

S.M.A.R.T. FITNESS PLAN	S.M.A.R.T. FOOD PLAN
Specific What activity(s) will I do? Time of day? (a.m. or p.m.) **M**easurable How many days will I exercise? Which days will I exercise? How many minutes will I do it for? **A**chievable Is this plan realistic? Reasonable? **R**elevant Is this an activity I enjoy? Can I make it a priority this week? **T**rackable Where will I record my activity?	**S**pecific What will I work on? **M**easurable How many days will I do it for? Which days will I target? (weekdays, weekends) **A**chievable Is this plan realistic? Reasonable? **R**elevant Will changing this eating habit make a difference in my health? **T**rackable How will I monitor this behavior?

Skill Practice: Week Nine

 As you grow more comfortable being in control of your weight and your health, practice planning for, instead of reacting to, people and situations that tend to derail your healthy intentions such as holidays, parties and food pushers. Focus on putting the skills needed to deal with these people or situations into motion this week.

1. **Keep records** —Keep track of your eating habits using one of the following methods. Check one option or create your own tracking system.

   ☐ Record food only.

   ☐ Record food and hunger/fullness cues.

   ☐ Use the Food Pyramid for a nutrition check. (See Appendix.)

   ☐ Record food and calories.

   ☐ Record food and fat grams.

   ☐ Record your feelings before each meal or snack.

   ☐ My own tracking system

   (specify): _____

2. **Practice being assertive** — Don't let others control your eating habits. Practice saying "No, thank you" to people who offer food when you don't feel hungry.

3. **Develop a plan for an upcoming celebration** — Follow through on the plan (page 222) you made for an upcoming event or celebration (holiday, birthday, party, etc.). Be sure to anticipate obstacles and plan some possible solutions to try.

4. **Put a new spin on your fitness routine** — Follow through with the activity you selected on page 223.

5. **S.M.A.R.T. plans** — Follow the fitness and food plans you made for yourself this week.

> *Reminder:* Don't forget to record your fitness activities in your FOOD & ACTIVITY JOURNAL.

FOOD & ACTIVITY JOURNAL

Date:_____

Day: M   Tu   W   Th   F   Sat   Sun

Fitness Activity:

TIME	FEELINGS CHECK	H/F SCALE*	FOOD & DRINK	AMOUNT	CALORIES	FAT (grams)	H/F SCALE*
					Total:	Total:	

*Rate your hunger/fullness on a scale from 0–10: 0 = Empty, 5 = Just Right, 10 = Stuffed

FOOD & ACTIVITY JOURNAL

Date:_____

Day: M   Tu   W   Th   F   Sat   Sun

Fitness Activity:

TIME	FEELINGS CHECK	H/F SCALE*	FOOD & DRINK	AMOUNT	CALORIES	FAT (grams)	H/F SCALE*
					Total:	Total:	

*Rate your hunger/fullness on a scale from 0–10: 0 = Empty, 5 = Just Right, 10 = Stuffed

FOOD & ACTIVITY JOURNAL

Date:_____

Day: M   Tu   W   Th   F   Sat   Sun

Fitness Activity: _____

TIME	FEELINGS CHECK	H/F SCALE*	FOOD & DRINK	AMOUNT	CALORIES	FAT (grams)	H/F SCALE*
					Total:	Total:	

*Rate your hunger/fullness on a scale from 0–10: 0 = Empty, 5 = Just Right, 10 = Stuffed

FOOD & ACTIVITY JOURNAL

Date:_____

Day: M   Tu   W   Th   F   Sat   Sun

Fitness Activity:

TIME	FEELINGS CHECK	H/F SCALE*	FOOD & DRINK	AMOUNT	CALORIES	FAT (grams)	H/F SCALE*
					Total:	Total:	

*Rate your hunger/fullness on a scale from 0–10: 0 = Empty, 5 = Just Right, 10 = Stuffed

FOOD & ACTIVITY JOURNAL

Date:_____

Day: M   Tu   W   Th   F   Sat   Sun

Fitness Activity:

TIME	FEELINGS CHECK	H/F SCALE*	FOOD & DRINK	AMOUNT	CALORIES	FAT (grams)	H/F SCALE*
					Total:	Total:	

*Rate your hunger/fullness on a scale from 0–10: 0 = Empty, 5 = Just Right, 10 = Stuffed

FOOD & ACTIVITY JOURNAL

Date:_____

Day: M Tu W Th F Sat Sun

Fitness Activity:

TIME	FEELINGS CHECK	H/F SCALE*	FOOD & DRINK	AMOUNT	CALORIES	FAT (grams)	H/F SCALE*
					Total:	Total:	

*Rate your hunger/fullness on a scale from 0–10: 0 = Empty, 5 = Just Right, 10 = Stuffed

FOOD & ACTIVITY JOURNAL

Date:_____

Day: M Tu W Th F Sat Sun

Fitness Activity:	

TIME	FEELINGS CHECK	H/F SCALE*	FOOD & DRINK	AMOUNT	CALORIES	FAT (grams)	H/F SCALE*
					Total:	Total:	

*Rate your hunger/fullness on a scale from 0–10: 0 = Empty, 5 = Just Right, 10 = Stuffed

Take Charge of Your Life

Congratulations—you've worked hard as a participant in the *Smart CHOICES* program. You've learned new skills and have begun to make positive changes in many aspects of your life. Your challenge in the weeks to come will be to continue applying the skills you've learned until they become an automatic part of your new lifestyle. This week you'll look at how far you've come and what you need to do next. Your continued success depends on having a plan for the future.

> ## This Week You Will:
>
> - Reflect over the previous week, noting insights and accomplishments.
> - Check the progress you've made during the program.
> - Prepare for dealing with lapses and learn how to prevent relapses.
> - Examine the components of a balanced lifestyle.
> - Review the "power" skills you now have in place.
> - Design a three-month S.M.A.R.T. plan to guide your future.

Reflections

 ### Reflect on your FOOD & ACTIVITY JOURNAL

Which aspect(s) of your food intake/eating patterns did you track? What did you learn from this activity?

Reflect on being assertive

Did you have any opportunities to turn down food during the past week? If yes, how did you handle it? What, if any, changes would you make in how you handled this situation?

Reflect on your skills for "surviving" celebrations

Did you have any opportunities to try some of the tips for eating in social situations? If yes, what techniques did you use?

Reflect on your S.M.A.R.T. plans

How did these plans work for you? Do you plan to use them again, throw them out or fine-tune them?

Other observations from last week

What worked well for you? What didn't work?

Facts of Life: Measuring Your Progress III

 Unless you had only a few pounds to lose, you most likely haven't reached your goal weight. As you know, that's OK. Slow weight loss is generally more permanent and easier to maintain. Be patient as you experiment with new tools and practice new skills. It takes six months to a year to turn new skills into new habits. If you continue to apply what you've learned, you will reach a healthy weight.

Take a few minutes to review the progress you've made over the course of this program. Check off the signs of success that you've experienced.

Healthier Eating Habits:

☑ I eat more fruits and vegetables.

☐ I eat more complex carbohydrates, such as whole grains and dried beans (legumes).

☑ I make lower-fat food choices.

☑ I plan ahead more often regarding meals and snacks.

☑ I eat smaller amounts.

Better Emotional Health:

☑ I pay more attention to my body's hunger/fullness signals (eat when hungry, stop before feeling stuffed).

☐ I no longer try to rigidly control my food by dieting.

☑ My attitude toward my body has improved (more respectful and accepting).

☐ I feel more at peace with food and the role it plays in my life.

☑ I am less critical of myself (less negative self-talk).

☐ I feel more capable of achieving and maintaining a healthier weight.

☐ I notice less emotional eating (I use food less often as a coping mechanism).

☐ I ask for support more often.

☑ I am more assertive in turning down food when I'm not hungry.

Improved Physical Health:

❑ I am more physically active on a regular basis.

❑ I've lost inches (body fat).

❑ I can climb stairs or carry packages more easily without getting short of breath.

❑ My clothes fit more comfortably.

❑ I am able to participate more fully in fun physical activities (such as hiking with the family).

❑ I have more energy throughout the day (fewer highs and lows).

❑ I move with greater ease.

Improved Medical Status:

❑ My blood sugars are under better control (improved diabetes control).

❑ My blood pressure is lower.

❑ My total cholesterol and/or LDL cholesterol level is lower.

❑ I am able to take less medication for a chronic health problem or illness.

Other Changes:

❑ _____

❑ _____

❑ _____

Reminder: Grab a tape measure and recheck the body measurements you took in Week One. Turn to page 14 and record your measurements.

Sense and Sensibility: Dealing with Lapses

 You've been exercising regularly for weeks now. You enjoy the energy it brings and notice that your clothes fit better. You leave on a week's vacation, and return to a jam-packed schedule. Before you know it, you haven't exercised in three weeks. Does this scenario sound familiar? It happens to everyone—an inevitable lapse, a time when you temporarily slip back into your old ways.

A lapse is simply a setback—a warning sign that your healthy habits have been derailed. Don't think of it as a catastrophe. Act immediately to prevent a lapse from turning into a relapse. If you fail to take action, you could "collapse" and revert back to old, unhealthy habits.

LAPSE →	**RELAPSE** →	**COLLAPSE**
happens once	happens more than once	means a return to old habits

Whether a lapse progresses to a relapse or a collapse depends on your response. If you lapse and slip into negative self-talk, you set yourself up for failure. On the other hand, if you acknowledge the lapse for what it represents, a temporary slip, you can move forward and get back on track.

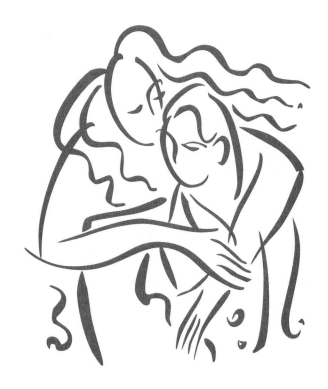

What to Do After a Slip-up

1. **Remain calm.** It's normal to feel guilty or want to blame someone after a lapse. Allow these feelings to rise up like a wave, peak and then pass away. Try not to react; just notice these feelings and let them pass. Forgive yourself and move on. No one is perfect.

2. **Speak gently to yourself.** Remind yourself that a lapse represents only a temporary setback. Even though you may feel out of control at the moment, you're not. You always have choices and options. Don't punish yourself when you temporarily slip back into old ways. Be aware of negative self-talk which can tempt you to throw in the towel. Do a reality check. Are your thoughts about your lapse realistic or distorted?

   Negative self-talk: *I blew it over the holidays. I've gained weight. I'll never get back in control.*

   Positive self-talk: *I've had a few weeks of backsliding. The holidays were tough. I'm ready to recommit to eating healthier and being more active. I'll stock the house with healthy foods and make arrangements with my walking partner.*

3. **Review the events leading up to a lapse or relapse.** Ask yourself the following questions: What events led up to the lapse? Were there any warning signs? What events took place during the lapse period? (Consider your mood, attitude, self-talk, setting and activities.)

   Example:

   - What events led up to the lapse?

     Preparing for the holidays, entertaining guests.

   - Were there any warning signs?

     Stopped exercising, didn't pay attention to what I ate, ignored hunger/fullness cues.

   - What events took place during the lapse period?

     Entertained house guests, didn't focus on healthy foods. Felt pressured to make all the traditional holiday goodies. Felt jovial—wanted to eat, drink and be merry.

4. **Learn from a lapse.** Look at a lapse as an opportunity for learning. Always ask yourself, "What did I learn from this experience and how can I handle things differently next time?"

Example:

- What did I learn from this experience?

   The holidays are a challenging time for me, especially if I'm entertaining guests.

- How can I handle things differently next time?

   It's easy to get off track during the holidays. Next time, I will incorporate a few lower-fat dishes into my meals. I'll plan in several walks during the week. I'll invite my guests to join me.

5. **Reaffirm your commitment.** After a lapse you may feel like giving up, like you've blown it. Think back over the reasons why you want to change your lifestyle. Are they worth giving up because you had this momentary setback? Remind yourself how far you've come and reflect back on past successes.

6. **Make a plan.** Set up a plan to counterbalance your slip that doesn't involve punishing yourself. Think about your previous recoveries and past successes. Be as specific as possible with your plan.

Example:

- Steps I will take to get back on track:

   At home, I will replace junk food with healthy foods I enjoy.

   I will enroll in a fitness class this week.

   I'll pack a healthy lunch for work three days this week.

7. **Talk to someone about your slip.** Seek out a friend, family member, group, class or health professional (dietitian, health educator, fitness specialist or counselor) for support and encouragement. If you can't talk to someone, write about it. Seeing it on paper can help clarify the situation.

Causes of Backsliding

When you slip up, stop and figure out why you lapsed. Understanding the reasons for slipping off track will help you avoid a relapse. What situations have gotten you off track in the past? What events triggered you to overeat or to stop your fitness program?

Researchers have identified several high-risk situations that could possibly derail your healthy intentions. Take a few minutes and check off the ones that might be triggers for you. Write down additional high-risk situations that come to mind.

Unpleasant emotions

❑ Anger

❑ Frustration

❑ Anxiety

❑ Boredom

❑ Depression

❑ Other:_____

Conflict with others

❑ Disagreement with a friend

❑ Argument with a spouse, child or other family member

❑ Disagreement with a manager or coworker

❑ Other:_____

Social pressure

❑ You eat because everyone else is eating.

❑ You drink because everyone else is having a cocktail.

❑ You're involved in holidays, parties, vacations or any other celebration involving food.

❑ You find it difficult to say no when others verbally pressure you to eat.

❑ Other:_____

Other high-risk situations (consider stress, workloads, relationships, etc.)

❑ Illness/injury

❑ Other:_____

❑ Other:_____

How to Prevent a Lapse

Select one of the high-risk situations you checked off in the previous section—a situation that has particular significance or special meaning for you. Take five to ten minutes to develop a plan for dealing with this situation in the future.

Example:

High-risk situation: Family gatherings are difficult. There is always so much food around. All we do is sit and eat.

Plan: Focus on fun instead of food. Plan in some fun activities for the next family event like badminton, croquet, volleyball or horseshoes.

Your High-Risk Situation:

Your Plan:

You are most likely to lapse when you find yourself unprepared for a situation. Plan ahead for high-risk situations. The more you can anticipate and plan ahead, the more confident you'll be.

Remember that a slip represents an opportunity to examine what went wrong and a way to prepare for the future. Think about an athlete—an Olympic ice skater, for example—who slips and falls many times on her way to success. Each time she falls, she consciously chooses to get up and continue rather than give up and call it quits.

The Balancing Act

Achieving a healthy lifestyle is a balancing act—it takes time and energy to be active, choose healthy foods, build supportive relationships, honor your feelings and emotions, and maintain positive self-talk. Creating a balanced lifestyle is easier said than done. What makes it so difficult to achieve? It takes commitment and hard work to make daily choices that support your priorities.

Unfortunately, our society doesn't value balanced living as much as it does a fast-paced schedule, a nice car, a big house or a prestigious career. You may feel like a fish swimming against the tide as you struggle to prioritize your time and make room for things that you feel are important—a yoga class, preparing a healthy meal or spending time in a meaningful relationship. You will need to be vigilant of the media and other cultural influences that constantly threaten to knock your priorities off balance.

What Do You Value?

Having a clear vision of your personal values sets the foundation for a balanced lifestyle. What is really important to you? Does your lifestyle reflect your values? If you say you value your health, yet you eat poorly, don't get enough rest, suppress your feelings and don't make time for fitness activities—do you really value your health?

What are your values? (Consider: family, adventure, knowledge, power, wealth, relationships, recognition, independence, security, creativity, beauty, health and helping others.)

List your personal values:

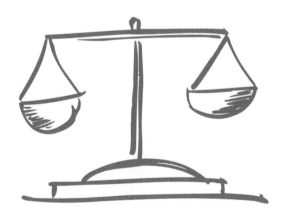

Does Your Time Reflect Your Values?

Do your current choices and behaviors match your values and beliefs? Take a few minutes to reflect on how you spend your time.

In the past week, what percentage of your time did you spend on each of the areas listed below? (Total should equal 100%.)

> *Note:* You may find that not all categories apply or that you need to add additional categories.

____ Self (personal time and growth)

____ Work (home and business)

____ Family

____ Fitness

____ Nutrition

____ Recreation, hobbies

____ Friends

____ Spiritual awareness (meditation, prayer, connection with nature, etc.)

____ Commitments (volunteer work, professional or organizational obligations, etc.)

____ Other: _____

____ Other: _____

How does the time spent in these areas compare with your values and your standards for success?

What, if any, changes would you like to make?

List one to three things you can do in the next three months to regain balance in your life.

Experiment to find the right balance. Each one of us defines and achieves balance in our own unique way. We all travel at our own pace. You may run well in high gear while someone else burns out at the thought of it. What constitutes balanced living for one person does not necessarily fit the bill for another.

The time and energy you invest in taking care of yourself and living a balanced life will pay off. You'll be healthier, decrease your risk for disease, develop quality relationships, and experience personal growth and a greater sense of well-being. It's in your hands —YOUR day-to-day choices determine the happiness and balance you experience in life.

Power On with Your New Skills

 The *Smart CHOICES* program contains many skills and techniques that were designed to help you achieve a healthier weight and lifestyle. Take five minutes to read through and check off all those you personally found helpful. Feel free to write in any that you do not find listed.

Skills and techniques that helped me

Monitoring and Planning

❑ Keeping a FOOD & ACTIVITY JOURNAL, monitoring _____.
(Food only, fat intake, calorie intake, hunger/fullness cues, feelings, exercise time).

❑ Designing weekly S.M.A.R.T. plans.

❑ Planning ahead for celebrations and holidays.

❑ Assessing my readiness for change (becoming more realistic in my decisions regarding change).

❑ Recognizing and tracking my progress beyond weighing myself on a scale.

Food/Nutrition

❑ Doing a reality check on portion sizes (e.g., weighing and measuring).

❑ Eating more fruits, vegetables and whole grains.

❑ Making lower-fat food choices.

❑ Allowing myself to eat in a balanced way without starving or depriving myself.

❑ Using information on food labels to guide my decisions about food choices.

❑ Using LIGHT, LEAN and LESS cooking techniques.

❑ Choosing lower-fat meals or smaller portions when eating away from home.

❑ Using the Food Pyramid to guide my food choices.

Emotional Health

❑ Seeking support or professional help when I need it.

❑ Paying attention to my body's hunger/fullness cues (eat when hungry, stop before feeling stuffed).

❑ Being more assertive in turning down food when I'm not hungry.

❑ Expressing my feelings and needs more often instead of stuffing them down with food. (Use food less often as a coping mechanism.)

❑ Challenging my inner critical voice about my weight and my body.

Fitness

☐ Exercising on a regular basis.

☐ Designing a workable fitness plan.

☐ Moving more in general (walking more, using stairs instead of the elevator, etc.).

Other Helpful Skills and Techniques

☐ _____

☐ _____

☐ _____

If you notice your weight creeping up or you start slipping back into old unhealthy habits, refer back to this list immediately. Figure out which skills or techniques you need to work on in order to regain control of your weight and your life.

Tips for Staying Motivated

- Challenge yourself by setting a goal that will move you into action. For example, a local fun-walk or hike might give you incentive to keep up your walking routine.

- Knowledge is power. Treat yourself to books or magazines that feature sound advice on nutrition, low-fat cooking, fitness, and tips for managing your weight.

- Reward or nurture yourself for the progress you have made. *Choose non-food rewards:* a massage or manicure, new book or magazine, listening to favorite music, craft/hobby projects, playing an instrument, flowers, a clean car, hot bubble bath, playtime with a pet, a long-distance phone call to someone special. See page 78 for more ideas.

- Chart your progress. Research tells us that you are more likely to stick with a behavior if you monitor it on a regular basis. Use whatever tool works for you: FOOD & ACTIVITY JOURNAL, fitness chart, calendar, daily planner, etc.

- Build support. Continue creating lines of support with family and friends. When that's not enough, consider support from a professional (dietitian, counselor, physician, fitness specialist or other health professional).

The Big Picture: A Three-Month S.M.A.R.T. Plan

 You've worked hard to learn new skills over the past couple of months. It takes time and practice for new skills to be transformed into new habits. The next three months are crucial to this process. Keep the following advice in mind as you continue—practice, practice, practice!

Stop and take ten to fifteen minutes to develop a S.M.A.R.T. plan for the next three months. Start by selecting three to five behaviors you want to work on during this period. These can be skills you wish to practice or new behaviors you'd like to try. Be as specific as possible.

Specific behaviors: Be precise about what you expect to achieve

EXAMPLE:	YOUR BEHAVIORS:
1. I will continue walking four days a week for 30 to 45 minutes per day.	1.
2. I will subscribe to a healthy cooking magazine.	2.
3. I will continue to write down what I eat five out of seven days a week.	3.
4. I will pack my lunch for work three days each week.	4.
5. I will continue to monitor my negative self-talk by writing it down in my diary. I'll then counter these thoughts with "balanced" self-talk.	5.

Measurable: What milestones will you use to measure your progress?

EXAMPLE:	YOUR BEHAVIORS:
1. Walk four days for 30 to 45 minutes.	1.
2. Try one new recipe each month.	
3. Record food intake five out of seven days.	2.
4. Pack lunch three out of five days.	3.
5. Record self-talk on weekday nights only.	4.
	5.

Achievable: Is your plan realistic given your schedule for the next three months?
Consider time constraints, commitments, time of year and available support. If after reviewing your plan you find it seems unreasonable, rework a more realistic one now.

Relevant: Will the behaviors you've chosen to work on make a difference in your health? What are the payoffs if you stick with them for three months?

Trackable: How will you track your progress?

EXAMPLE:	YOUR BEHAVIORS:
1. Record in my daily planner.	1.
2. Expand my collection of healthy, low-fat recipes.	
3. Record in my FOOD & ACTIVITY JOURNAL.	2.
4. Record in my FOOD & ACTIVITY JOURNAL.	3.
5. Write in my personal diary.	4.
	5.

Building Support for Yourself

As you continue your journey toward a healthier weight and lifestyle, a little moral support can go a long way. Support comes in various forms:

- Family members supporting your efforts to eat healthy

- A friend who's committed to walking with you regularly

- A class or program—fitness, cooking, yoga, assertiveness, dance, etc.

- Therapist or program specializing in issues around emotional eating

- Books and magazines—walking, fitness, body acceptance, nutrition, etc.

- A personalized consultation with a dietitian or fitness trainer

- Giving yourself a mental pat on the back for positive actions

- Rewarding yourself in ways that don't involve food

Think about the behaviors you want to work on. What type of support would be most useful? Write down several ways you can enlist support for yourself over the next three months.

The Journey: Not the End, Just a Rest Stop

In the past weeks, you've gained powerful skills and new insight into your health behaviors. With time and practice, these new health behaviors will become an automatic part of your lifestyle. Remember, it's the small choices you make day to day—ordering a veggie pizza instead of "the works"; leaving the table feeling satisfied, not stuffed; going for a walk instead of watching TV—that add up in the long run.

Acknowledge your progress. Few things are as powerful as your own feelings of self-pride. Nurture this pride by giving yourself credit for present and past successes. Be quick to give yourself a pat on the back and slow to scold yourself. Don't hold back and wait for big changes such as a drop in clothing size. Instead, notice and acknowledge the smaller positive choices that you make every day.

There will be setbacks—it's part of the process. You now have the skills to work through rough times. You can speak to yourself in an encouraging voice, make a S.M.A.R.T. plan, and ask for help. This workbook will always be there for you. Each time you reread it, you'll glean another helpful nugget.

Take care of your body—feed it well, move it, rest and nurture it. You are given only one body in your lifetime. You can't trade it in or make an exchange, so nourish and nurture the body you have.

You are not on a diet but on a journey toward better health. There are no time pressures, no right or wrong ways. Each path is a new learning experience, each person's journey a unique adventure. This is not the end, just a rest stop along the way. Best wishes for a happy, healthy future!

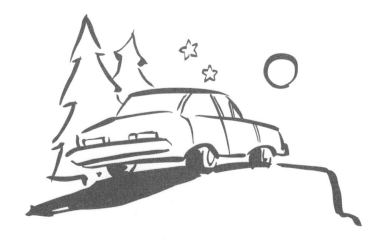

Appendix

CALORIE & FAT COUNTER

Contents:

Beverages
Dairy and Eggs
Fats and Oils
Fish and Shellfish
Fruit
Grains and Pasta
Meats: Beef, Game, Lamb, Pork, Lunch Meats
Nuts and Seeds
Poultry
Salad bar foods
Sauces and Dips
Snack Foods
Soups
Sweets
Vegetables
Restaurant Foods
Fast Foods

This CALORIE & FAT COUNTER represents a small selection of food items listed in alphabetical order. Check food labels for the most accurate calorie and fat information. Use this counter when food label information is unavailable. Many books and websites provide more extensive food listings. Listed below are three are several resources that might be useful:

Harriet Roth's Fat Counter by Harriet Roth, second edition. Signet books, 1999. This book lists calories, fat, percentage of calories from fat, cholesterol, saturated fat and sodium counts for thousands of foods.

Fast Food Facts: The Original Guide for Fitting Fast Food into a Healthy Lifestyle by Marion Franz, fifth edition. International Diabetes Center, 1998. Order through http://www.amazon.com or NCES (800) 445-5653. This book features nutrition information on 40 popular restaurants.

Olen Publishing— http://www.olen.com/food This website features a food finder that contains 1200 food items from 25 fast food restaurants.

FOOD	AMOUNT	CALORIES	FAT (grams)
Beverages			
Alcoholic			
Beer	12 oz	150	0
Egg nog	8 oz	342	19
Hard liquor (gin, rum, vodka, whiskey) 80-90 proof	1.5 oz	95-110	0
Wine	4 oz	80-85	0
Carbonated			
Club soda	12 oz	0	0
Soft drinks	12 oz	125-160	0
Coffee drinks			
(If topped with whipped cream, add 60 calories and 5 grams of fat.)			
Caffe Mocha, nonfat milk	8 oz	155	11
Caffe Mocha, 2% milk	8 oz	175	13
Caffe Mocha, whole milk	8 oz	195	15
Caffe Latte, nonfat milk	8 oz	68	1
Caffe Latte, 2% milk	8 oz	90	4
Caffe Latte, whole milk	8 oz	114	6
Cappuccino	8 oz	100	5
Coffee	8 oz	5	0
Sports drinks			
All Sport	8 oz	70	0
Gatorade	8 oz	50	0
Powerade	8 oz	70	0
Other Beverages			
Cocoa			
With whole milk	6 oz	135	6
With nonfat milk	6 oz	90	0
Fruit drinks, canned or bottled	6 oz	80-100	0
Tea	8 oz	0	0

FOOD	AMOUNT	CALORIES	FAT (grams)
Dairy and Eggs			
Cheese			
American	1 oz	106	9
Blue	1 oz	100	8
Brie	1 oz	90	8
Cheddar	1 oz	114	10
Colby	1 oz	112	9
Cottage cheese			
4% fat	1/2 cup	110	5
2% fat	1/2 cup	102	2
1% fat	1/2 cup	90	1
Cream cheese			
Fat Free	2 Tbsp (1 oz)	30	0
Light (1/3 less fat)	2 Tbsp (1 oz)	70	6
Regular	2 Tbsp (1 oz)	100	10
Feta	1 oz	75	6
Gouda	1 oz	101	8
Gruyere	1 oz	117	9
Monterey Jack	1 oz	106	9
Mozzarella			
Whole milk	1 oz	80	6
Shredded	1 oz	90	7
Part skim	1 oz	72	5
Parmesan	1 Tbsp	23	2
Provolone	1 oz	100	8
Ricotta			
Whole milk	1/2 cup	216	16
Part skim	1/2 cup	171	10
Romano	1 oz	110	8
Swiss	1 oz	107	8
Cream			
Light, coffee or cooking	1 Tbsp	29	3
Sour cream			
Regular	1 Tbsp	30	3
Light	1 Tbsp	18	1
Whipping cream			
Fluid	1 cup	821	88
Whipped	1/2 cup	205	22
Non-dairy (Cool Whip Lite)	2 Tbsp	20	1

FOOD	AMOUNT	CALORIES	FAT (grams)
Dairy and Eggs (Continued)			
Milk			
Skim	1 cup	85	Trace
1% fat	1 cup	102	2.5
2% fat	1 cup	122	5
Whole	1 cup	160	10
Buttermilk	1 cup	100	2
Chocolate			
2% fat	1 cup	180	5
Whole	1 cup	210	8
Condensed, sweetened	1 Tbsp	65	1.5
Evaporated			
Skim	1 cup	200	1
Whole	1 cup	340	19
Yogurt			
Low-fat, all brands	8 oz	120-250	2-3
Nonfat, all brands	8 oz	110-190	0
Egg			
Whole, large	1 egg	75	5
White	1 white	16	0
Yolk	1 yolk	61	5
Egg substitute	1/4 cup	30-40	0-1
Fats and Oils			
Butter	1 Tbsp	108	12
Margarines			
Regular	1 Tbsp	100	11
Light	1 Tbsp	50	6
Mayonnaise			
Regular	1 Tbsp	100	11
Reduced calorie	1 Tbsp	50	5
Oils	1 Tbsp	120	13
Shortening, Crisco	1 Tbsp	110	12

FOOD	AMOUNT	CALORIES	FAT (grams)
Fish and Shellfish			
Clams			
Breaded and fried	20 small	379	21
Raw, cherrystone	20 small	133	2
Cod	3 oz	90	1
Crab, Alaska King	3 oz	81	2
Flounder	3 oz	99	2
Haddock	3 oz	96	1
Halibut	3 oz	120	3
Lobster	3 oz	84	1
Mussels, blue	3 oz	72	1
Octopus, raw	3 oz	69	1
Oysters, raw	1 med	41	1
Roughy, Orange	3 oz	108	2
Salmon			
Raw, Atlantic	3 oz	120	5
Pink, canned	3 oz	117	5
Sardines, canned in oil, drained	2 sardines	50	3
Scallops	3 oz	96	2
Shrimp			
Raw	4 lg	30	2
Breaded and fried	4 lg	73	4
Snapper	3 oz	108	2
Sole	3 oz	99	2
Swordfish	3 oz	132	5
Trout	3 oz	129	4
Tuna			
Solid white in water	3 oz	120	1.5
Solid white in oil, drained	3 oz	165	9

Fruit

60 calories and 0 grams of fat.

Fruit

Apple, 1 small (4 oz)
Applesauce, unsweetened, 1/2 cup
Apples, dried, 4 rings
Apricots, fresh, 4 whole (5 1/2 oz)
Apricots, dried, 8 halves
Apricots, canned, 1/2 cup
Banana, small, 1 (4 oz)
Blackberries, 3/4 cup
Blueberries, 3/4 cup
Cantaloupe, 1 cup cubes
Cherries, fresh, 12 (3 oz)
Cherries, sweet, canned, 1/2 cup
Dates, 3
Figs, fresh, 2 medium (3 1/2 oz)
Figs, dried, 1 1/2
Fruit cocktail, 1/2 cup
Grapefruit, 1/2 large
Grapefruit sections, 3/4 cup
Grapes, small, 17 (3 oz)
Honeydew melon, 1 cup cubes
Kiwi, 1
Mandarin oranges, canned, 3/4 cup
Mango, 1/2 small
Nectarine, 1 small
Orange, 1 small
Papaya, 1/2 fruit or 1 cup cubes
Peach, 1 medium fresh or 1/2 cup canned
Pear, 1/2 fresh or 1/2 cup canned
Pineapple, 3/4 cup fresh or 1/2 cup canned
Plums, 2 small or 1/2 cup canned
Prunes, 3 dried
Raisins, 2 Tbsp
Raspberries, 1 cup
Strawberries, 1 1/4 cup
Tangerines, 2 small (8 oz)
Watermelon, 1 1/4 cup cubes

Fruit Juice

Apple juice/cider, 1/2 cup
Cranberry juice cocktail, 1/3 cup
Cranberry juice cocktail, reduced-calorie, 1 cup
Fruit juice blends, 100% juice, 1/3 cup
Grape juice, 1/3 cup
Grapefruit, 1/2 cup
Orange juice, 1/2 cup
Pineapple juice, 1/2 cup
Prune juice, 1/3 cup

FOOD	AMOUNT	CALORIES	FAT (grams)
Grains and Pasta			
Breads			
Bagels	4 oz	310	1-2
Biscuits	1 biscuit	200	7-10
Bread sticks	5 sticks	120	2-4
Challah	1" slice	160	4
Croissant	1 (2 oz)	230	12
Croutons	2 Tbsp	30	1
English muffin	1 muffin	120	1
French bread	2" slice	130	0
French toast	1 slice	140	8
Garlic bread	1 slice (2 oz)	190	8
Muffins, most varieties	4.5 oz	400	11
Multi-grain bread	1 slice	160	2
Oatmeal bread	1 slice	60	1
Pita bread			
White	1 piece	150	1
Whole-wheat	1 piece	180	1
Pumpernickel bread	1 slice	80	1
Raisin bread	1 slice	80	1
Rolls			
Hamburger and hot dog	1 roll	120	2
Hard rolls	1 roll	160	1
Hoagie	1 roll	200	4
Rye bread	1 slice	80	1
Sourdough bread	1 slice	130	1
White bread	1 slice	65-100	1-2
Whole-wheat bread	1 slice	65-100	1-2
Cereals, Cold			
Cold cereals vary widely in their calorie content (55-400 calories per cup) and fat content (0-20 grams per cup). Check food labels for exact values.			

FOOD	AMOUNT	CALORIES	FAT (grams)
Grains and Pasta (Continued)			
Cereals, Hot			
Cream of Rice	1 cup	127	0
Cream of Wheat	1 cup	133	0
Malt-O-Meal	1 cup	120	0
Oatmeal	1 cup	145	2
Oat Bran	1 cup	170	3
Ralston	1 cup	135	1
Wheatena	1 cup	136	1
Grains			
Couscous, cooked, no added fat	1 cup	190	0.5
Rice, cooked, no added fat			
Brown	1 cup	200	2
White	1 cup	227	0
Wild	1 cup	166	0
Pastas			
All types, dry	2 oz	210	1
Chow mein noodles	1/3 cup	140	7
Ravioli, chicken	1 cup	330	12
Tortellini			
Chicken	1 cup	290	10
Cheese	1 cup	300	9
Mixed Pasta Dishes			
Fettuccini Alfredo	1 cup	880	68
Spaghetti w/ meatballs	1 cup	270	10
Italian Rigatoni	1 cup	320	12
Macaroni and cheese	1 cup	410	19
Meats: Beef, Game, Lamb, Pork, Lunch Meats—Cooked Portions			
Beef, cooked			
Arm pot roast	3 oz	297	22
Bottom round steak	3 oz	222	12
Brisket	3 oz	348	30
Chuck steak	3 oz	324	26

FOOD	AMOUNT	CALORIES	FAT (grams)
Flank steak, trimmed	3 oz	210	10
Ground beef, 20% fat	3 oz	228	15
Ground beef, 15% fat	3 oz	204	12
Ground beef, 10% fat	3 oz	170	9
Porterhouse steak	3 oz	255	18
Rib roast	3 oz	324	25
Rump roast	3 oz	294	23
Shortribs	3 oz	400	35
Sirloin steak, trimmed	3 oz	200	10
T-bone steak	3 oz	276	21
Tenderloin steak, trimmed	3 oz	203	12
Top round	3 oz	180	7
Veal cutlet, no breading	3 oz	186	9
Game & Organ Meat			
Rabbit, stewed	3 oz	174	7
Brain, simmered	3 oz	135	11
Liver	3 oz	138	4
Lamb			
Chop, loin	3 oz	306	25
Cubed lamb, lean	3 oz	160	6
Ground lamb	3 oz	243	17
Leg	3 oz	220	16
Rib	3 oz	306	25
Shoulder, whole	3 oz	290	21
Pork			
Chop, loin, trimmed	3 oz	172	7
Chop, rib, trimmed	3 oz	186	8
Roast, loin, trimmed	3 oz	165	6
Roast, rib, trimmed	3 oz	182	9
Shoulder cut, picnic	3 oz	282	23
Spareribs	3 oz	340	26
Tenderloin, lean, trimmed	3 oz	140	4

FOOD	AMOUNT	CALORIES	FAT (grams)
Meats (Continued)			
Sausages and Lunch Meats			
Bologna, beef	1 oz	90	8
Frankfurter, beef	2 oz	190	17
Frankfurter, chicken	2 oz	120	11
Frankfurter, turkey	2 oz	110	8
Ham, baked, lean	1 oz	34	1.5
Kielbasa, pork, beef	2 oz	180	17
Pepperoni, regular	1 oz	140	13
Pepperoni, turkey	1 oz	80	4
Salami, beef	1 oz	73	6
Sausage, beef	2 oz	212	20
Turkey breast, processed	1 oz	35	.5
Turkey ham	1 oz	40	2
Nuts and Seeds			
Nuts			
Almonds	1 oz	165	15
Cashews	1 oz	163	13
Coconut, shredded	1 oz	101	10
Peanuts, shelled	1 oz	161	14
Peanut butter	1 Tbsp	95	8
Pecans	1 oz	187	18
Pistachio	1 oz	172	15
Walnuts	1 oz	182	18
Seeds			
Sesame			
Regular	1 Tbsp	47	4
Tahini	1 Tbsp	90	8
Sunflower	1 oz	170	16
Poultry			
Chicken			
Breast, roasted, skinless	3 oz	140	3
Breast, fried, batter-dipped	3 oz	220	11
Leg, roasted, skinless	3 oz	162	7
Leg, fried, batter-dipped	3 oz	225	13
Thigh, roasted, skinless	3 oz	178	9
Thigh, fried, batter-dipped	3 oz	232	14
Wing, roasted	1	100	7
Wing, fried, batter-dipped	1	160	11

FOOD	AMOUNT	CALORIES	FAT (grams)
Duck			
Roasted, meat only	3 oz	170	10
Turkey			
Dark meat, roasted, skinless	3 oz	160	6
Light meat, roasted, skinless	3 oz	135	3
Ground, fresh	3 oz	180	10
Ground, fresh, breast	3 oz	110	1
Salad Bar Foods			
Bacon bits	1 Tbsp	105	3
Breadsticks	2 sticks	20	<1
Cheddar, shredded	1/4 cup	110	9
Chow mein noodles	1/2 cup	140	7
Cottage cheese	1/2 cup	110	5
Croutons	2 Tbsp	30	1
Olives			
Green	4 med	15	2
Black	3 sm or 2 lg	15	2
Salads			
Cole slaw	1/2 cup	180	12
Macaroni	1/2 cup	280	18
Potato	1/2 cup	180	10
Three bean	1/2 cup	130	2
Tuna	1/2 cup	190	9
Sunflower seeds	1 oz	170	16
Sauces and Dips			
Sauces			
Barbecue	2 Tbsp	50	1
Béarnaise	2 Tbsp	106	11
Cheese	2 Tbsp	62	5
Cream	2 Tbsp	56	5
Curry Cream	2 Tbsp	80	7
Hollandaise	2 Tbsp	164	18
Horseradish	1 Tbsp	20	2
Louis	2 Tbsp	126	13
Marinara	1/2 cup	100	4
Nacho cheese	2 Tbsp	90	7
Pesto	1/4 cup	310	30

FOOD	AMOUNT	CALORIES	FAT (grams)
Sauces and Dips (Continued)			
Sauces			
Soy	1 Tbsp	11	0
Tartar	1 Tbsp	70	8
White	2 Tbsp	48	4
Worcestershire	1 Tbsp	0	0
Dips			
French onion	2 Tbsp	60	5
Green onion	2 Tbsp	50	5
Guacamole	2 Tbsp	50	3
Hummus with tahini	2 Tbsp	57	3
Salsa	2 Tbsp	12	0
Snack Foods			
Chips, Crisps, etc.			
Cheetos	21 pieces	150	9
Fritos	32 chips	160	10
Potato chips	15-22 chips	150	10
Potato sticks	3/4 cup	160	10
Pretzels	1 oz	110	1
Sun Chips, Multigrain	11 chips (1 oz)	140	6
Tortilla chips	7-15 chips	140	7
Crackers			
Cheese Nips	29 pieces	150	7
Goldfish	55 pieces	140	7
Hearty wheat	13	140	6
Matzo	1 piece	110	2
Oysterettes	19 pieces	60	2
Ritz	5	80	4
Saltines	5	60	2
Sociables	7	80	4
Town House	5	80	4
Triscuit wafers	7	140	5
Waverly	5	70	3
Wheatsworth	5	80	3
Popcorn			
Air-popped	1 cup	30	0
Movie Theater			
In oil	sm (7 cups)	398	27
In oil with "butter"	sm (7 cups)	632	50

FOOD	AMOUNT	CALORIES	FAT (grams)
Soups			
Chicken noodle	1 cup	70	3
Cream of mushroom	1 cup	170	17
French onion	1 cup	350	14
Minestrone	1 cup	90	2
New England clam chowder	1 cup	230	16
Vegetable	1 cup	70	3
Sweets			
Cakes			
Angel Food	1/12 cake	125	0
Carrot	1/8 cake	350	21
Cheesecake	1/12 cake	280	18
Crumb coffee	1/10 cake	250	12
Cupcake	1 cupcake	340	15
Decorated sheet	1 slice (3 oz)	320	18
Devil's food	1 slice (3 oz)	360	19
Fruit cake	1 slice (4.5 oz)	470	19
German chocolate	1/16 cake	521	31
Pound	2" slice	300	16
Candy			
Creme de menthe	8 thins (1.4 oz)	200	12
Caramels	4 pieces (1.3 oz)	150	4
Hard candies	1 oz	110	0
Hershey's Kisses	8 (1.4 oz)	210	12
Milk chocolate			
Plain	1 bar (1.5 oz)	230	13
With almonds	1 bar (1.5 oz)	230	14
Licorice sticks	4 (1.3 oz)	140	0
M & M's	1 bag (1.8 oz)	230	10
Peanut brittle	1.4 oz	180	4
Yogurt-covered nuts	11 (1.5 oz)	210	13
Frozen Yogurt			
TCBY			
Small	5 oz	163	4
Medium	7 oz	228	6
Large	9 oz	293	8

FOOD	AMOUNT	CALORIES	FAT (grams)
Sweets (Continued)			
Ice Cream			
Premium ice cream	1/2 cup	230-320	14-24
Light ice cream	1/2 cup	100-150	1-5
Dove bars	1 bar	270	17
Ice cream sandwich	1	170	6
Pies			
Fruit	1/6 pie (4 oz)	280	14
Cream/Custard	1/4 pie (5 oz)	410	22
Pecan	1/6 pie (4 oz)	440	22
Puddings			
Chocolate mousse	1/2 cup	324	22
Creme caramel	1 cup	303	14
Custard, baked	1 cup	305	7
Cookies			
Biscotti	1 (1 oz)	270	2
Brownie	2" square	140	7
Chocolate chip	1 (1 oz)	140	7
Gingersnap	5 (1 oz)	130	4
Oatmeal	1 (1 oz)	110	3
Oreo			
Regular	3 (1 oz)	160	7
Reduced fat	3 (1 oz)	130	3.5

Vegetables

25 calories and 0 grams of fat per 1/2 cup cooked or one cup raw.

(If margarine or butter is added, add 100 calories and 11 grams of fat per tablespoon.)

Artichokes
Asparagus
Beans (green, wax, Italian)
Bean sprouts
Beets
Broccoli
Brussels sprouts
Cabbage
Cauliflower
Celery
Cucumber
Eggplant
Green onions
Greens (collard, kale, mustard, turnip)
Kohlrabi
Leeks
Mushrooms
Okra
Onions
Pea pods
Peppers (all varieties)
Radishes
Salad greens (endive, escarole,
    lettuce, romaine, spinach)
Sauerkraut
Spinach
Summer squash
Tomato
Tomatoes, canned
Tomato sauce
Tomato/vegetable juice
Turnips
Water chestnuts
Zucchini

Starchy Vegetables:
80 calories and 1 gram of fat.

Baked Beans, 1/3 cup
Corn, 1/2 cup
Corn on cob, 1 medium (5 oz)
Mixed vegetables with corn and peas, 1 cup
Peas, green, 1/2 cup
Plantain, 1/2 cup
Potato, baked or boiled, 1 small (3 oz)
Potato, mashed, 1/2 cup
Squash, winter (acorn, butternut), 1 cup
Yam, sweet potato, 1/2 cup

FOOD	AMOUNT	CALORIES	FAT (grams)
Restaurant Food			
Chinese Restaurant			
Hors d'oevres			
Egg rolls	1 egg roll	152	12
Soups			
Hot and sour soup	1 serving	165	8
Wonton soup	1 serving	283	12
Entrées			
Beef			
With any vegetable(s)	1 dish	1572	119
Kung Pao beef	1 dish	2458	190
Orange beef	1 dish	1710	135
Chicken			
With cashews	1 dish	1765	119
With any vegetable(s)	1 dish	1224	72
Kung Pao chicken	1 dish	1806	126
Pork			
With any vegetable(s)	1 dish	1574	135
Barbecued (not fried)	1 dish	1374	110
Moo Shu pork	1 dish	1383	117
Spareribs, barbecues	1 dish	1863	137
Sweet and sour	1 dish	1845	168
Szechaun	1 dish	1694	149
Shrimp			
Hunan (not deep-fried)	1 dish	1068	84
Kung Pao shrimp	1 dish	1068	84
Sweet and sour	1 dish	1069	89
International House of Pancakes (IHOP)			
Pancakes			
Buttermilk	1 (2 oz)	108	3
Buckwheat	1 (2.25 oz)	134	5
Waffles			
Regular	1 (4 oz)	305	15
Belgian, regular	1 (6 oz)	408	20

FOOD	AMOUNT	CALORIES	FAT (grams)
Italian Restaurant			
Appetizers			
Antipasta	1.5 lbs	629	47
Entrées			
Fettucine Alfredo	2.5 cups	1498	97
Lasagna	2 cups	958	53
Linguine			
With red clam sauce	3 cups	892	23
With white clam sauce	3 cups	907	29
Spaghetti			
With meat sauce	3 cups	928	25
With meatballs	3.5 cups	1155	39
With tomato sauce	3.5 cups	849	17
Veal parmigiana with spaghetti	1.5 cups	1064	44
Side Dishes			
Fried calamari	3 cups	1037	70
Garlic bread	1 piece (2 oz)	190	8
Spaghetti with tomato sauce	1.5 cups	409	8
Mexican Restaurant			
Appetizers			
Beef and cheese nachos *	1 serving	1362	89
Cheese quesadilla *	1 serving	900	59
Cheese nachos	1 serving	807	56
Entrées			
Beef burrito *†	1 serving	1639	79
Beef chimichanga *†	1 serving	1607	86
Beef enchilada †	2 enchiladas	1253	58
Chicken fajitas and flour tortilla *†	1 serving	1661	63
Chile rellenos †	2 rellenos	1578	96
Chicken enchilada †	2 enchiladas	1264	57
Crispy chicken taco †	2 tacos	1042	42
Taco salad	1 serving	1099	71
*With sour cream and guacamole †With beans and rice			

FOOD	AMOUNT	CALORIES	FAT (grams)
Restaurant Food (Continued)			
Mexican Restaurant			
Side Dishes			
Rice	3/4 cup	229	4
Refried beans	3/4 cup	375	16
Tortilla chips	50 chips	645	48
Sandwiches (restaurant or sandwich shop)			
Bacon, lettuce and tomato	8 oz	599	37
Chicken salad			
Plain bread	10 oz	537	32
With mayo	10 oz	655	46
Corned beef with mustard	9 oz	497	20
Egg salad with mayo	10 oz	664	44
Grilled cheese	5 oz	511	33
Ham			
With mustard	9 oz	563	27
With mayo	9 oz	666	40
Reuben	14 oz	916	50
Roast beef			
With mustard	9 oz	462	12
With mayo	9 oz	565	24
Tuna salad with mayo	11 oz	833	56
Turkey			
With mustard	9 oz	370	6
With mayo	9 oz	473	19
Turkey club	13 oz	737	34
Vegetarian	12 oz	753	40

FOOD	AMOUNT	CALORIES	FAT (grams)
Submarine Sandwiches (Subway)			
BMT			
Plain bread	6 inch	491	28
With mayo or oil	6 inch	609	44
Cold cut combo			
Plain bread	6 inch	379	16
With mayo or oil	6 inch	497	29
Ham and cheese			
Plain bread	6 inch	322	9
With mayo or oil	6 inch	440	22
Meatball	6 inch	444	39
Roast beef			
Plain bread	6 inch	345	12
With mayo or oil	6 inch	463	25
Spicy Italian			
Plain bread	6 inch	522	32
With mayo or oil	6 inch	640	45
Steak and cheese	6 inch	371	13
Tuna salad			
Plain bread	6 inch	551	36
With mayo or oil	6 inch	669	49
Turkey			
Plain bread	6 inch	308	9
With mayo or oil	6 inch	426	22
Veggies and cheese			
Plain bread	6 inch	272	9
With mayo or oil	6 inch	389	22

FOOD	AMOUNT	CALORIES	FAT (grams)
Fast Foods			
Arby's			
Baked potato			
Plain	1	355	0
Broccoli 'n cheese	1	571	20
Chicken broccoli	1	841	56
Biscuit, plain	1	280	15
Croissant			
Plain	1	220	12
Sausage and egg	1	520	39
Chicken club sandwich	1	546	31
Chicken deluxe sandwich, grilled	1	430	31
Curly Fries			
Cheddar	1	333	18
Regular	1	300	10
Ham 'n Swiss sub sandwich	1	500	23
Horsey sauce	1 Tbsp	60	5
Light sandwiches			
Roast beef deluxe	1	296	10
Roast chicken deluxe	1	276	6
Roast turkey deluxe	1	260	7
Jr. Roast Beef	1	324	14
Regular	1	388	19
Super	1	523	27
Giant	1	555	28
Burger King			
BK Big Fish Sandwich	1	720	43
BK Broiler Chicken Sandwich	1	530	26
BK Broiler Chicken Sandwich w/o mayo	1	370	9
Chicken Sandwich	1	710	43
Chicken Sandwich w/o mayo	1	500	20
Chick'N Crisp Sandwich	1	460	27
Chicken Tenders	5 pieces	230	14
Coca Cola Classic, medium	22 oz	280	0
Croissan'wich with Sausage, Egg & Cheese	1	530	41
Dutch apple pie	1	300	15

FOOD	AMOUNT	CALORIES	FAT (grams)
Dipping sauces			
Barbecue	1 oz	35	0
Honey flavored	1 oz	90	0
Honey mustard	1 oz	90	6
Ranch	1 oz	170	17
Sweet and sour	1 oz	45	0
Shakes, medium, all flavors	14 oz	440	10
French Fries			
Small	1	250	13
Medium	1	400	21
King size	1	590	30
Onion Rings			
Medium	1	380	19
King size	1	600	30
Whopper Sandwich	1	660	40
With Cheese	1	760	48
Double Whopper Sandwich	1	920	59
With Cheese	1	1010	67
Whopper Jr. Sandwich	1	400	24
With Cheese	1	450	28
Hamburger	1	320	15
Cheeseburger	1	360	19
Bacon Cheeseburger	1	400	22
Double Cheeseburger	1	580	36
Bacon Double Cheeseburger	1	620	38
Dairy Queen			
Banana Split	1	510	12
Blizzard			
Chocolate sandwich cookie, small	10 oz	520	18
Chocolate sandwich cookie, medium	12 oz	640	23
Breeze			
Strawberry, small	10 oz	320	.5
Strawberry, medium	14 oz	460	1
Cone			
Vanilla, small	5 oz	230	7
Vanilla, medium	7 oz	330	9
Vanilla, large	9 oz	410	12

FOOD	AMOUNT	CALORIES	FAT (grams)
Fast Foods (Continued)			
Dairy Queen			
Cone, dipped			
Small	6 oz	340	17
Medium	8 oz	490	24
DQ Sandwich	1	150	5
Misty Slush			
Small	16 oz	220	0
Medium	21 oz	290	0
Peanut Buster Parfait	1	730	31
Shake, chocolate			
Small	14 oz	560	15
Medium	19 oz	770	20
Sundae, chocolate, medium	1	400	10
Yogurt, medium cup	7 oz	230	.5
Dunkin' Donuts			
Donuts			
Apple fritter	1	300	14
Eclair	1	270	11
Glazed cruller	1	290	14
Jelly filled	1	210	8
Old fashioned cake type	1	250	16
Yeast (glazed)	1	180	8
Muffins			
Apple 'N Spice	1	350	12
Blueberry	1	320	12
Blueberry, low-fat	1	250	1
Bran, low-fat	1	240	1
Honey Raisin Bran	1	390	12
Kentucky Fried Chicken (KFC)			
Original recipe chicken sandwich	1	497	22
Mashed potatoes with gravy	1	120	6
Extra Tasty Crispy			
Breast	1	470	28
Drumstick	1	190	11
Thigh	1	370	25
Wing	1	200	13

FOOD	AMOUNT	CALORIES	FAT (grams)
Hot & Spicy			
Breast	1	530	35
Drumstick	1	190	11
Thigh	1	370	27
Wing	1	210	15
Original recipe			
Breast	1	276	14
Drumstick	1	150	9
Thigh	1	290	21
Wing	1	181	12
Tender Roast			
Breast (with skin)	1	251	11
Drumstick (with skin)	1	112	6
Thigh (with skin)	1	207	12
Wing (with skin)	1	121	8
McDonald's			
Big Mac	1	560	31
Cheeseburger	1	320	13
Chicken McNuggets	6 piece	290	17
Chicken salad deluxe	1	120	1.5
Egg McMuffin	1	290	12
Filet O Fish	1	450	25
Fries			
Small	1	210	10
Large	1	450	22
Super size	1	540	26
Grilled Chicken Deluxe	1	440	20
Hamburger	1	260	9
Hash brown potatoes	1	130	8
Quarter Pounder	1	420	21
With cheese	1	530	30
Salad dressings			
Caesar	2 oz	160	14
Fat-free Herb Vinaigrette	2 oz	50	0
Ranch	2 oz	230	21
French, reduced calorie	2 oz	160	8
Sausage McMuffin	1	360	23

FOOD	AMOUNT	CALORIES	FAT (grams)
Fast Foods (Continued)			
McDonald's			
Desserts/Shakes			
Apple pie	1	260	13
McFlurry, M & M	1	630	35
Shakes, all flavors	14 oz	360	9
Sundae, hot fudge	1	340	18
Pizza Hut			
Hand-tossed pizza, medium			
Cheese	2 slices	618	18
Pepperoni	2 slices	602	16
Super supreme	2 slices	718	24
Supreme	2 slices	666	22
Pan pizza, medium			
Cheese	2 slices	722	30
Pepperoni	2 slices	706	28
Super supreme	2 slices	802	36
Supreme	2 slices	770	34
Personal pan pizza			
Pepperoni	1 pizza	810	28
Supreme	1 pizza	808	27
Taco Bell			
Border Wraps			
Steak Fajita	1	470	21
Chicken Fajita	1	460	20
Veggie Fajita	1	420	19
Steak Supreme	1	510	25
Chicken Supreme	1	520	26
Veggie Supreme	1	510	24
Burritos			
Bean	1	380	12
Burrito Supreme	1	440	19
Chicken	1	400	14
Chicken Burrito Supreme	1	500	20
Gorditas, Fiesta			
Beef	1	290	13
Chicken	1	260	10
Steak	1	270	10

FOOD	AMOUNT	CALORIES	FAT (grams)
Gorditas, Santa Fe			
Beef	1	380	20
Chicken	1	370	20
Steak	1	370	10
Gorditas, Supreme			
Beef	1	300	13
Chicken	1	300	14
Steak	1	310	14
Tacos			
Taco	1	180	10
Soft Taco	1	220	10
Taco Supreme	1	220	14
Soft Taco Supreme	1	260	14
Steak Soft Taco	1	230	10
Chicken Soft Taco	1	200	7
Specialty Items			
Tostado	1	300	15
Mexican Pizza	1	570	35
Taco Salad	1	850	52
Taco Salad without shell	1	420	22
Cheese Quesadilla	1	350	18
Nachos	1	320	18
Beef Nachos Supreme	1	450	24
Pintos 'N Cheese	1	190	9
Wendy's			
Baked potato			
Plain	1	310	0
Broccoli & cheese	1	470	14
Cheese	1	570	23
Chili & cheese	1	630	24
Sour cream & chives	1	380	6
Big Bacon classic	1	580	30
Chicken club sandwich	1	470	20
Cheeseburger, Jr.	1	320	13
Chili			
Small	1	190	6
Large	1	290	9
Frosty dairy dessert, small	1	330	8

FOOD	AMOUNT	CALORIES	FAT (grams)
Fast Foods (Continued)			
Wendy's			
Hamburgers			
Plain single	1	360	16
Single with everything	1	420	20
Junior	1	270	10
Grilled Chicken Sandwich	1	310	8
French fries			
Small	1	270	13
Biggie	1	470	23
Fresh Salads			
Grilled chicken salad	1	200	8
Side salad	1	60	3
Fresh Stuffed Pitas			
Chicken Caesar	1	490	18
Classic Greek	1	440	20
Garden Veggie	1	400	17

Surviving a Snack Attack without a Fat Attack

Fruit

- Fresh, frozen, canned or baked
  Ideas: baked apple, broiled grapefruit, frozen grapes, bananas or raisins
- Fruit leather or roll-ups (without added sugar)
- Dried fruit

Veggies

Carrots, celery sticks, green pepper rings, broccoli, jicama, cauliflower, cucumber slices, mushrooms, radishes. Serve with your favorite low-fat dip or salad dressing.

Dairy Products

Reduced-fat cheeses (6 grams of fat or less per ounce)
- Laughing Cow (light)
- String cheese
- Low-fat cottage cheese

Nonfat or low-fat yogurt — layer with fruit and low-fat granola for a parfait or blend with frozen fruit and frozen juice concentrate for a smoothie.

Grains

Bagels *
Breads (any kind; whole grain
   varieties are more nutritious)
Breadsticks
Crackers, low-fat (4 grams of fat or less per ounce)
Chips (3 grams of fat or less per ounce)
Muffins* (5 grams of fat or less per muffin)
Popcorn (air-popped or light microwave brands)

Popcorn cakes
Pretzels—hard and soft varieties
Rice Cakes
Tortillas

Cereals (low sugar varieties), some examples:

Cheerios	Raisin Bran**
Cornflakes	Rice Krispies
Puffed Rice, Corn, Wheat	Shredded Wheat**

*   Large bagels and muffins may contain as many as 500-600 calories.
** Higher fiber

Frozen Treats
(Look for brands that are 0-2 grams of fat per 1/2 cup serving)

- Light ice cream
- Nonfat or low-fat frozen yogurt
- Fruit juice bars
- Fudgesicles

Beverages

- Coffee latté, nonfat
- Herbal tea
- Hot cocoa (low-fat packaged varieties or cocoa mixed with nonfat milk)
- Milk, nonfat or 1%
- Mineral & seltzer waters (unsweetened)

Breakfast Ideas

- Whole grain bagel spread with fat-free or light cream cheese.

- Nonfat yogurt topped with fresh fruit and/or cereal (e.g., Grapenuts or low-fat granola).

- Hot or cold cereal with skim or 1% milk.

- Whole grain toast or English muffin spread with a thin layer of peanut butter and jam.

- Pancakes or waffle topped with applesauce, jam, syrup, flavored yogurt, or powdered sugar. Make your favorite recipe and lower the fat, or try a low-fat store brand.

- Fruit smoothie — blend low-fat yogurt or milk with fresh, canned or frozen fruit (berries, peaches or bananas). Sweeten with a dash of vanilla extract and frozen juice concentrate.

- Low-fat cottage cheese with fruit and whole grain toast or bagel.

- Breakfast sandwich — two slices whole grain toast, a thin slice of warmed lean ham or turkey ham, and an egg (or egg substitute) cooked in a non-stick skillet with vegetable oil spray.

- Bran, whole grain or fruit muffin (5 grams of fat or less per muffin; in baking, use one teaspoon of fat or less per muffin) and a glass of low-fat milk.

- Skinny Hash Browns — slice leftover baked or roasted potatoes and cook in a non-stick skillet with vegetable oil spray. Add chopped onion and green pepper. Season with garlic powder, basil or oregano and add a sprinkle of Parmesan cheese.

- Reduced-fat cheese (6 grams of fat or less per ounce) melted on a slice of whole grain toast.

Tip: For a nutrition boost, add a glass of 100% juice, a sprinkle of dried fruit, or a piece of fresh fruit to your breakfast.

Lunch Ideas

Use these suggestions as the basis for a healthy lunch. Add bread, crackers, milk, fruit or vegetables as needed.

- Burritos — spread a flour tortilla with refried beans, roll up and wrap in plastic. Include salsa to spoon on when ready to eat. (Tip for packers or brown baggers: package the beans separately to avoid sogginess.)

- Baked potato topped with low-fat cottage cheese or reduced-fat cheddar cheese, and green onions or chives. (Tip for packers: put toppings in plastic containers or zip lock bags.)

- Soup (vegetable, noodle, lentil or bean) with crackers or bread sticks.

- Nonfat yogurt, a whole grain bagel and a piece of fruit.

- Tossed salad, fresh vegetable salad or bean salad in pita bread with low-fat salad dressing. (Tip for packers: put salad in a container with the dressing at the bottom. Just before eating, shake container to mix the dressing with the other ingredients and assemble pita sandwich.)

- Fruit salad: low-fat cottage cheese or yogurt with fruit and a hard roll.

- Laughing Cow Light cheese wedges spread on a bagel or low-fat crackers.

- Pasta with meatless spaghetti sauce. Vary the sauce and try different types of pasta, such as angel hair, rigatoni, etc.

- Leftovers reheated in a microwave: rice or pasta dishes, vegetables, potatoes, soup, etc.

- Reconstituted low-fat dehydrated soups or ramen noodles. Serve with crackers and a piece of fruit. (*Note:* These soups tend to be high in sodium.)

Pointers for Packers

- Foods containing eggs, meat or dairy products need to be refrigerated or packed in an insulated bag with a frozen ice pack.

- Good finger-vegetables: cherry tomatoes, baby carrots, radishes, cauliflower, broccoli, jicama, celery.

- To prevent soggy sandwiches, pack lettuce, sliced tomatoes and cucumbers separately and add them to your sandwich immediately before eating.

- Low-fat sandwich filling ideas: turkey breast, tuna with nonfat or low-fat mayo, turkey ham, lean ham, turkey pastrami, mashed beans (e.g., hummus), veggie burgers, low-fat cheese, light or nonfat cream cheese.

- Low-fat sandwich spread ideas: mustard, horseradish, catsup, cranberry sauce, relish, cocktail sauce, chutney, nonfat or low-fat mayonnaise.

- Bored with bread? Try corn or flour tortillas, rice cakes, crackers, bagels, pita bread, muffins, bread sticks or rolls.

Lowfat & Fast Recipes

The following recipes have been reprinted with permission from the cooking video, *LOWFAT & FAST! . . . Real Food for Busy People*™ by Becker & Miller, 1996.

Beef Stir Fry With Rice

Makes 4 servings

6 cups cooked rice

Sauce ingredients:
   3/4 cup hot water
   1/2 teaspoon beef bouillon base (*or* 1/2 cube)
   2 tablespoons reduced-sodium soy sauce
   2 tablespoons seasoned rice vinegar
   1 rounded tablespoon cornstarch

Vegetable oil spray
12 ounces beef sirloin, sliced in thin strips
1 teaspoon sesame oil
1/2 – 1 tablespoon *fresh* ginger root, grated
1/2 – 1 tablespoon garlic, minced
1 cup celery, chopped
1 red pepper, sliced
1 cup pea pods
1 can (5 oz.) sliced water chestnuts, drained

Start cooking rice.

Combine sauce ingredients in a small bowl.

Spray a non-stick skillet or wok with vegetable oil spray and sauté beef strips until barely done. Remove beef and set aside. Measure sesame oil into wok and add ginger and garlic. Add celery and red pepper, cook 1 minute. Add pea pods and water chestnuts, followed by the sauce and beef strips. Cook two minutes longer allowing sauce to bubble and thicken.

Serve over hot rice.

- 530 calories, 5 grams fat, 480 mg. sodium per serving.
- About 1 1/2 cups stir fry with 1 1/2 cups rice per serving.

Variations:
Substitute chicken, turkey tenderloin, halibut, shrimp, scallops, pork loin or tofu in place of beef. Any combination of vegetables will work. Experiment with your favorite veggies. To save time and keep fresh ginger root fresh, chop in food processor and freeze in small container.

Pasta With Black Beans & Corn

Makes 4 servings
3 cups cooked rotini pasta (6 ounces dried)
Vegetable oil spray
1 teaspoon garlic, minced (or 1/2 tsp. garlic powder)
1/2 cup onion, chopped
1 can (15 oz.) chopped stewed tomatoes, undrained
1 can (15 oz.) black beans, rinsed and drained
1 can (15 oz.) corn kernels, drained
1/2 – 1 tablespoon chili powder
2 teaspoons cumin
1 teaspoon oregano

Cook pasta, drain and set aside.

Spray a large pot with vegetable oil spray, sauté garlic and onion until tender. Stir in tomatoes, bean, corn, chili powder, cumin and oregano. Bring to a boil, reduce heat and simmer for 5 minutes, stirring occasionally. Add pasta to bean mixture in pot, toss gently and heat thoroughly.

- 360 calories, 2 grams fat, 500 mg. sodium per serving.
- About 1 1/2 cups per serving.

Baked Herbed Fish With Rice

Makes 4 servings
6 cups cooked rice
1 1/2 pounds fish fillets
1 tablespoon cooking oil
1 teaspoon thyme leaves
Pinch of salt or Lite salt
2 cloves garlic, minced
1/2 cup onion, chopped
1 cup white wine or skim milk (not both)
Sprinkle of paprika (optional)

Start cooking rice.

Preheat oven to 400 degrees.

Place fish fillets in baking dish. Combine oil with thyme, salt and garlic. Spread over fish. Top with onions. Pour wine (*or* skim milk) over the fish. Bake for 10-15 minutes or until fish flakes with a fork.

Serve with rice, using the pan juices as sauce.

- 580 calories, 6 grams fat, 445 mg. sodium per serving.
- Approximately 4 oz. fish with 1 1/2 cups rice per serving.

Pasta With Clam Sauce

Makes 4 servings
5 cups cooked pasta (about 12 ounces dried)
2 cans (10 oz.) *whole* baby clams, undrained
1 teaspoon garlic, minced
Juice of one large lemon (*or* 1 cup white wine)
2 tablespoons olive oil
1 cup chopped fresh parsley (optional)

Cook pasta, drain and set aside.

In a small saucepan combine all ingredients except the pasta. Heat until just boiling.

Pour over hot pasta and serve.

- 320 calories, 8 grams fat, 315 mg. sodium per serving.
- About 1 1/2 cups per serving.

Variations:
Substitute 2 cans (6 oz. each) of albacore tuna packed in water for the clams.

Black Beans With 100 Uses

Makes 4 servings
2 cans black beans, rinsed and drained
1 cup water
1/2 cup onion, chopped
2 cloves garlic, minced
1 teaspoon brown sugar
1 tablespoon cumin
1 teaspoon oregano
2 bay leaves, broken in half
Pinch salt or Lite salt
1/4 cup freshly squeezed lemon juice
2 – 3 drops Tabasco sauce

Place all ingredients in a saucepan and cook over medium heat for 20 minutes.

Black Beans with 100 Uses can be stored in the refrigerator for several days; simply heat and serve.

- 165 calories, 1 gram fat, 500 mg. sodium per serving.
- 1 cup per serving.

Just a few of the 100 uses...
- Burritos, tacos, or taco salad
- Served over rice and topped with salsa
- Served over pasta
- Dilute with water for Black Bean Soup (puree, if you like it smooth)
- Try them with low-fat tortilla chips and low-fat grated cheese for nachos

Chicken Pécante With Rice

Makes 4 servings
6 cups cooked rice
4 boneless, skinless chicken breasts (16 ounces)
Vegetable oil spray
3/4 cup fresh salsa
1/3 cup Dijon mustard
Juice of 1 lemon

Start cooking rice.

Cut chicken into two-inch cubes.

Spray a non-stick skillet with vegetable oil spray. Heat skillet and sauté chicken cubes until browned (about 10 minutes, depending on thickness). Meanwhile, combine salsa, mustard and lemon juice. Pour over chicken and simmer for 2 or 3 minutes until sauce is heated and chicken is completely cooked.

Serve over rice.

- 530 calories, 4 grams fat, 510 mg. sodium per serving.
- 3 oz. chicken with 1 1/2 cups rice per serving.

Focaccia Pizza

Makes 4 servings
Focaccia bread
1 cup low-fat or fat-free spaghetti or marinara sauce
2 tablespoons grated Parmesan cheese
1 1/2 cups (6 oz.) shredded skim milk, Lite or fat-free mozzarella cheese

Preheat oven to 400 degrees.

Cut focaccia bread into 2 flat circles. Place cut side up on baking sheet. Spread each half with about 1/2 cup of the spaghetti sauce. Sprinkle each half with 1 tablespoon of the Parmesan and 3/4 cup shredded mozzarella cheese.

Bake for 15-20 minutes until cheese is melted.

- 429 calories, 9 grams fat, 1290 mg. sodium per serving (if made with skim milk mozzarella cheese).
- 384 calories, 3 grams fat, 1338 mg. sodium per serving (if made with fat-free mozzarella cheese).
- One-fourth total recipe per serving.

Variations:
Try different breads for the "crust" such as thawed frozen bread dough, pita bread or French bread.

Try vegetable toppings such as green or red peppers, steamed broccoli, mushrooms, onions or artichoke hearts (packed in water).

Small amounts of flavorful meats can be used. Try smoked turkey, Canadian bacon, lean ham, turkey ham or turkey pepperoni.

Chicken Fajitas

Makes 4 servings

12 ounces boneless, skinless chicken breasts

8 low-fat flour tortillas

Seasoning marinade:

   1 tablespoon chili powder

   2 teaspoons cumin

   1 tablespoon Worcestershire sauce

   2 tablespoons balsamic vinegar

   1 tablespoon water

Vegetable oil spray

1 small onion, sliced

1 green or red pepper, sliced

2 tablespoons nonfat sour cream, or plain yogurt

2 tablespoons salsa

Cut chicken into long thin strips. Warm tortillas in oven (wrap in foil) or microwave (cover with damp towel). Combine seasoning marinade in a bowl, add chicken strips. Marinate chicken while slicing onion and pepper. Sauté onion and pepper in oil-sprayed skillet until cooked but still crisp, remove from pan. Add chicken and sauté for 2-3 minutes until done. Add onion/pepper mixture and leftover marinade. Cook an additional minute. Add a little water if too dry.

Fill warm tortillas with chicken, top with nonfat sour cream or yogurt and salsa.

- 330 calories, 7 grams fat, 470 mg. sodium per serving.
- 2 fajitas per serving.

Red Beans And Rice

Makes 4 servings

6 cups cooked rice

Vegetable oil spray

1/2 cup onion, chopped

1 can (14.5 oz.) Cajun-flavored stewed tomatoes

2 cans red beans (15 oz. each) rinsed and drained

1 can (4 oz.) diced green chilies

3 – 6 drops Tabasco sauce

Start cooking rice.

Coat a medium sized pot with vegetable oil spray, sauté onion until tender. Add stewed tomatoes, beans, chilies, and Tabasco sauce. Cover and simmer for 10 minutes.

Serve over a bowl of cooked rice.

- 530 calories, 1 gram fat, 650 mg. sodium per serving.
- 1 1/4 cups beans with 1 1/2 cups rice per serving.

Pasta Primavera

Makes 4 servings
5 cups cooked pasta (about 12 ounces dried)
1 tablespoon olive oil
1/2 cup onion, chopped
2 garlic cloves, minced
3 – 4 cups broccoli florets and stems
1/2 chicken bouillon cube
1/2 cup water
1/2 cup white wine
1/2 cup freshly grated Parmesan cheese
Fresh ground pepper to taste
1 teaspoon red pepper flakes (optional)

Cook pasta, drain and set aside.

In a large skillet, sauté onion and garlic in olive oil. Add broccoli to pan and sauté for 1 minute. Add bouillon cube, water and wine, and stir until broccoli is bright green and bouillon has dissolved.

Combine with pasta and top with Parmesan cheese, pepper and red pepper flakes, if desired.

- 390 calories, 9 grams fat, 345 mg. sodium per serving.
- About 2 cups pasta with sauce per serving.

Variations:
Can be made with asparagus, zucchini, mustard greens or any combination of vegetables in place of broccoli.

Selected Resources

Books

Behavior & Attitude Changes

Changing for Good by James Prochaska, John Norcross and Carlo DiClemente. Avon Books, 1994.

Coping with a Negative Body Image by Kathy Bowen-Woodward. The Rosen Group, 1989.

Women's Comfort Book: A Self-Nurturing Guide for Restoring Balance in Your Life by Jennifer Louden. HarperCollins, 1992.

Fitness

ACSM Fitness Book by The American College of Sports Medicine, Second edition. Human Kinetics, 1998.

Great Shape: The First Fitness Guide for Large Women by Pat Lyons and Debby Burgard. Bull Publishing, 1990.

Strong Women Stay Young by Miriam Nelson. Bantam Books, 1997.

Non-dieting Approaches to Food and Weight

Intuitive Eating: A Recovery Book for the Chronic Dieter by Evelyn Tribole and Elyse Resch. St. Martin's Press, 1995.

Making Peace with Food: Freeing Yourself from the Diet/Weight Obsession by Susan Kano. Harper-Row, 1989.

The Solution: Winning Ways to Permanent Weight Loss by Laurel Mellin. HarperCollins, 1997.

Thin for Life: Ten Keys to Success from People Who have Lost Weight & Kept It Off by Anne Fletcher. Firefly Books Ltd, Ontario, Canada, 1994.

When Food is Love: Exploring the Relationship between Eating & Intimacy by Geneen Roth. Penguin Books, 1991.

When Women Stop Hating Their Bodies: Freeing Yourself from the Food and Weight Obsession by Jane Hirschmann and Carol Munter. Fawcett, 1995.

You Count, Calories Don't (2nd ed.) by Linda Omichinski. Tamos Books, Winnipeg, Canada, 1999.

Cookbooks

Cooking Light Cookbooks. Oxmoor House, (800) 633-4910. http://www.cookinglight.com

For Goodness' Sake: An Eating Well Guide to Creative Low-Fat Cooking. Camden House Publishing, Inc., 1990.

Moosewood Restaurant Cooks at Home: Fast & Easy Recipes for any Day, Moosewood Collective. Simon & Schuster, 1994.

New Dieters Cookbook, Better Homes and Gardens. Meredith Books, 1992

Pasta Light: Over 200 Great Tasting Low Fat Pasta Recipes. Time Life Books, 1998.

Quick & Healthy Recipes & Ideas (Volumes I & II) by Brenda Ponichtera. Scale Down Publishing, 1519 Hermits Way, The Dalles, OR 97058, (541) 296-5859, 1995.

Sunset Low Fat Cookbooks. Sunset Publishing Corporation, 80 Willow Road, Menlo Park, CA 94025, (800) 634-3095.

Tastefully Oregon. Oregon Dietetic Association, P.O. Box 6497, Portland, OR 97228, 1996.

The Best 125 Low Fat Fish & Seafood Dishes by Susann Geiskopf-Hadler and Mindy Toomary. Prima, 1993.

The Best 125 Vegetable Dishes by Susann Geiskopf-Hadler and Mindy Toomary. Prima, 1994.

The New American Diet Cookbook by Sonja Connor and William Connor. Simon & Schuster, 1997.

The Vegetarian Way by Virginia Messina and Mark Messina. Harmony Books, 1996.

Newsletters and Magazines

Berkeley Wellness Letter, P.O. Box 420148, Palm Coast, Florida 32142, (904) 445-6414.

Big Beautiful Woman, P.O. Box 458, Mt. Morris, IL 61054-9806, (800) 707-5592.

Cooking Light: The Magazine of Food and Fitness, Circulation Department, Box 1748, Birmingham, AL 35201, (800) 336-0125. http://www.cookinglight.com

Environmental Nutrition: The Newsletter of Diet, Nutrition & Health, P.O. Box 420451, Palm Coast, FL 32142-0451, (800) 829-5384.

Lipid Clinic News, L465, OHSU, 3181 SW Sam Jackson Park Road, Portland, OR 97201, (503) 494-7775.

Nutrition Action Healthletter, Center for Science in Public Interest, 1501 16th Street, Washington D.C. 20836, (800) 237-4874. http://www.cspinet.org

Radiance: The Magazine for Large Women, P.O. Box 30246, Oakland, CA 94604, (510) 482-0680. http://www.radiancemagazine.com

Tufts University Health and Nutrition Letter, P.O. Box 57843, Boulder, CO 80321-7843, (800) 274-7581. http://www.navigator.tufts.edu

Videos

Body Trust: Undieting Your Way to Heatlh and Happiness by Dayle Hayes, 2110 Overland Avenue, Suite 120, Billings, MT 59102, (800) 321-9499, 1994. One hour video.

Lowfat & Fast!...Real Food for Busy People by Nancy Becker & Sandy Miller, P.O. Box 69611, Portland, OR 97201, (503) 977-9868, 1996. Thirty-five minute cooking video.

For exercise videos, call for *The Complete Guide to Exercise Videos* catalog at (800) 433-6769. Exercise videos are reviewed and rated by fitness level and exercise type (aerobics, muscle toning, stretching, mind-body).

Websites

American Dietetic Association http://www.eatright.org Accurate food and nutrition information provided by a professional association of dietitians.

Consumer Information Center http://www.pueblo.gsa.gov Education materials on health, food and nutrition which have been reviewed and published by government agencies.

Cyberdiet http://www.cyberdiet.com Interactive site that allows viewers to seek help and share successes with others striving to lose weight.

Healthy Weight Journal http://www.healthyweight.net Current scientific articles on eating and weight.

Mayo Health Oasis http://www.mayohealth.org Sponsored by Mayo Clinic, good source of nutrition information and advice you can trust.

Meals For You http://www.mealsforyou.com Hundreds of recipes that can be sorted by type, ingredient, nutrient content or special needs.

Nutrition Links http://www.oznet.ksu.edu Covers age-specific information, sites for specific medical conditions, vegetarian diets and general health pages.

Obesity and Weight Control from Michael Myers, MD http://www.weight.com Dr. Meyers answers questions on weight loss and obesity, covering gimmicks and treatment options.

Phys. http://www.phys.com Chat rooms, forums, rate your diet, calculators that calculate body mass index, caloric needs, and target heart rate.

Shape Up America http://www.shapeup.org Provides current information on safe weight management, healthy eating, and physical fitness.

Tufts University Nutrition Navigator http://www.navigator.tufts.edu Reviews and rates on-line nutrition sites.

USDA Food & Nutrition Information Center http://www.nal.usda.gov/fnic Information on the Food Guide Pyramid; electronic copies of the Pyramid.

WIN: Weight Control Information Network http://www.niddk.nih.gov Collection of reliable articles on obesity and weight loss from the National Institutes of Health.

Professional Resources

Moving Away From Diets: New Ways to Heal Eating Problems & Exercise Resistance by Karin Kratina, Nancy King & Dayle Hayes. Helm Seminars, Publishing, P.O. Box 1295, Lake Dallas, TX 75065, (817) 497-3558, 1996. Book.

Weight Management Facilitator Training Program: How to Guide Others Through the Process of Change by Greg Phillips & Gail Johnston. SOF Publishing, 98 Everett Drive, Suite C, Durango, CO 81301, (800) 869-6393, 1995. Six-tape audiocassette home-study course.

FOOD & ACTIVITY JOURNAL

Date:_____

Day: M Tu W Th F Sat Sun

Fitness Activity:

TIME	FEELINGS CHECK	H/F SCALE*	FOOD & DRINK	AMOUNT	CALORIES	FAT (grams)	H/F SCALE*
					Total:	Total:	

*Rate your hunger/fullness on a scale from 0–10: 0 = Empty, 5 = Just Right, 10 = Stuffed

Your Personal Food Pyramid

Fats, Oils, Sweets

Milk Products
(2–3 servings)

1. _____
2. _____
3. _____

Meat & Alternatives
(2–3 servings)

1. _____
2. _____
3. _____

Vegetables *(3–5 servings)*

1. _____
2. _____
3. _____
4. _____
5. _____

Fruits *(2–4 servings)*

1. _____
2. _____
3. _____
4. _____

Breads, Cereals, Rice, Pasta *(6–11 servings)*

1. _____   5. _____   9. _____
2. _____   6. _____   10. _____
3. _____   7. _____   11. _____
4. _____   8. _____

What changes do you plan to make? _____

_____

_____

_____

EMOTIONAL EATING: TAKING BACK CONTROL WORKSHEET

Step 1. Identify Your Feelings

What are you feeling? It's possible to feel more than one emotion at a time. Write them all down. Use I FEEL statements.

Step 2. Use Feelings to Identify Your Needs

Your feelings will help you identify what you need. Write down possible ways of meeting these needs without food.

Step 3. Make Effective Requests: Communicate Your Feelings and Needs

After you identify your feelings and your needs, you may want to use this information to make a request. (In some cases, you may identify what you need from yourself as well as from others.) Communicate your feelings using an I FEEL statement.

Step 4. Identify Attitudes and Beliefs That Get in the Way

Be alert to any attitudes that undermine your well-being. List any attitudes and beliefs that may become obstacles to getting your needs met.

Order Form

To order your *Smart CHOICES for Health*™ workbooks, complete this form and send with a check, credit card number or purchase order number to:

Attn: *Smart CHOICES*
Providence Resource Line
Tigard Business Center
11308 SW 68th Parkway, Suite 125
Tigard, OR 97223
www.providence.org/classes

Make checks payable to: Providence Health System
Quantity discounts: 20% discount on orders of 10 or more + Shipping and Handling.

☐ Send me information on the *Smart CHOICES for Health*™ Instructor Guide.

☐ I want to order _____ *Smart CHOICES for Health*™ workbooks at $24.95 each $ _____

Shipping and Handling at $3.00 each $ _____

TOTAL ENCLOSED = $ _____

Payment Method

☐ **Check**

☐ **Credit Card:** **Visa** **MasterCard** **Discover**

Card # _____

Exp. Date _____ / _____ Signature _____

☐ **Purchase Order #** _____

Bill to:
Name _____
Dept/Org _____
Street _____
City _____ St _____ Zip _____
Phone: (_____) _____

Ship to:
Name _____
Dept/Org _____
Street _____
City _____ St _____ Zip _____
Phone: (_____) _____

Office Use only:
Order date: Shipping method: Invoice #:
Billing date: Ship date: